Activity
Analysis
& Application

FOURTH EDITION

Activity Analysis & Application

FOURTH EDITION

Nancy K. Lamport, MS, OTR
Indiana University School of Medicine
Indianapolis, Indiana

Margaret S. Coffey, MA, COTA, ROH
LaPorte, Indiana

Gayle I. Hersch, PhD, OTR
School of Occupational Therapy
Texas Woman's University
Houston, Texas

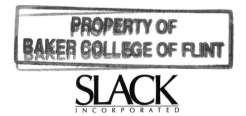

SLACK
INCORPORATED

an innovative information, education, and management company

6900 Grove Road • Thorofare, NJ 08086

Publisher: John H. Bond
Editorial Director: Amy E. Drummond
Senior Associate Editor: Jennifer Stewart

The procedures and practices described in this book should be implemented in a manner consistent with the professional standards set for the circumstances that apply in each specific situation. Every effort has been made to confirm the accuracy of the information presented and to correctly relate generally accepted practices. The author, editor, and publisher cannot accept responsibility for errors or exclusions or for the outcome of the application of the material presented herein. There is no expressed or implied warranty of this book or information imparted by it. Any review or mention of specific companies or products is not intended as an endorsement by the author or the publisher.

The work SLACK publishes is peer reviewed. Prior to publication, recognized leaders in the field, educators, and clinicians provide important feedback on the concepts and content that we publish. We welcome feedback on this work.

Lamport, Nancy K.
    Activity Analysis & Application / Nancy K. Lamport, Margaret S. Coffey, Gayle I. Hersch.--4th ed.
        p. ; cm.
    Includes bibliographical references and index.
    ISBN 1-55642-487-6 (alk. paper)
    1. Occupational therapy--Handbooks, manuals, etc. I. Title: Activity analysis and application. II. Coffey, Margaret S., III. Hersch, Gayle Ilene. IV. Title.
        [DNLM: 1. Occupational Therapy--methods. 2. Occupational Therapy--organization & administration. 3. Outcome and Process Assessment (Health Care)--organization & administration. 4. Task Performance and Analysis. WB 555 L238ab 2001]
    RM735.3 .L35 2001
    615.8'515--dc21

                                                                                        00-066119

Printed in the United States of America

Published by: SLACK Incorporated
                   6900 Grove Road
                   Thorofare, NJ 08086 USA
                   Telephone: 856-848-1000
                   Fax: 856-853-5991
                   www.slackbooks.com

    Last digit is print number: 10 9 8 7 6 5 4 3 2 1

CONTENTS

INSTRUCTORS: *Activity Analysis & Application, Fourth Edition Instructor's Manual* is also available from SLACK Incorporated. Don't miss this important companion to this textbook. To order the *Instructor's Manual*, please contact SLACK Incorporated at 856-848-1000. Or visit us on the web at www.slackbooks.com.

ACKNOWLEDGMENTS

The authors wish to acknowledge all those who have helped us in our long-term study of activity analysis and its application to occupational therapy intervention. We have learned from our students and from each other. We have sought and received feedback from our colleagues, and we have flourished under the never-failing guidance and support of our editors and friends at SLACK Incorporated. In this, the Fourth Edition, John Bond, vice president of book publishing; Amy Drummond, editorial director; Debra Toulson, managing editor; and Jennifer Stewart, senior associate editor, have again remained but an email or phone call away.

We are grateful to our husbands and children for the many times they momentarily managed our usual assigned roles when deadlines closed in. We appreciate the opportunity to be a part of a profession that encourages growth and scholarship among its members and has given us the confidence to grow intellectually, professionally, and personally. We are grateful to each other for the forbearance we seem to have maintained through four editions of this material and still remain friends as well as co-authors. It is in this spirit of support, growth, and respect that we dedicate this Fourth Edition of *Activity Analysis & Application*.

Nancy K. Lamport, MS, OTR
Margaret S. Coffey, MA, COTA, ROH
Gayle I. Hersch, PhD, OTR

ABOUT THE AUTHORS

Nancy K. Lamport, MS, OTR

Ms. Lamport is associate professor emerita with the Occupational Therapy Program, School of Allied Health Sciences, Indiana University School of Medicine, Indianapolis. She teaches part-time in the area of leisure skills and serves as alumni coordinator for the Occupational Therapy Program.

Margaret S. Coffey, MA, COTA, ROH

Ms. Coffey is a former lecturer with the Occupational Therapy Program, School of Allied Health Sciences, Indiana University School of Medicine, Indianapolis. She practiced in long-term care facilities serving the geriatric population until 1999. Currently, she is a freelance writer and is teaching occupational therapy concepts in handspinning and weaving activities to the well population.

Gayle I. Hersch, PhD, OTR

Dr. Hersch is an associate professor in the School of Occupational Therapy at Texas Woman's University—Houston Center. Her responsibilities are in the areas of teaching and research with master's and doctoral students. Major course content includes adult development and gerontology; performance areas, components, and contexts; and qualitative research. Prior to joining the faculty at Texas Woman's University—Houston Center in 1994, she was on faculty for 11 years in the Occupational Therapy Program, School of Allied Health Sciences, Indiana University School of Medicine, Indianapolis.

PREFACE

This is the Fourth Edition of *Activity Analysis Handbook* and reflects ongoing growth in this essential area of our academic and professional knowledge base. When we began work in this area in 1983, instructional materials were drafted primarily to fill a void in the classroom. Forms were developed to bridge the gap in student learning regarding the importance of activity and the use of activity in occupational therapy. Seventeen years later, these forms, with minor changes, are still intended to facilitate the student's understanding of what is involved in performing an activity and how using that activity with a given client makes a difference. Regardless of the therapist's frame of reference, theoretical background, or method of treatment, a thorough knowledge of activity and its potential use in therapy is needed. In this book, the authors guide students through a thought process to the point of discerning meaningful, purposeful activities for use in occupational therapy intervention.

In this edition, the text has been divided into Modules and Units to facilitate the learning of more in-depth material in specific areas. There are additions and expansions to incorporate new information from literature reviews, to clarify material used in previous editions, and to present relevant ideas that have emerged since the last revision. The Activity Analysis Form has been separated into two sections to aid in learning. An *Instructor's Manual* is now available, which contains much of the original Chapter Four and student examples of completed forms from Chapter Three. Information on downloading the blank forms from our companion website is also provided.

Uniform Terminology for Reporting Occupational Therapy Services, first published in 1979, has also undergone three revisions during the years of its use, and additional changes have been made to this material recently. In 1999, *The Guide to Occupational Therapy Practice* was introduced as an additional way of more closely focusing the ramifications of practice and documentation.

The authors' premise remains that all activities used in occupational therapy can be recorded in Uniform Terminology. In this text, Uniform Terminology provides a unifying framework for working through the material and forms presented. The ability to document the use and importance of purposeful activity is the goal for every student. For this reason, the First and Third Editions have been retained as appendices to aid the student in completing the forms and understanding the definitions of terms used in practice.

Several changes in terms reflect the incorporation of the most current usage in the American Occupational Therapy Association (AOTA) document *The Guide to Occupational Therapy Practice* (1999). The term "practitioner" replaces "therapist" and refers to both occupational therapists and occupational therapy assistants. The term "intervention" replaces the more limited concept implied by the word "treatment." The term "independent function" continues to be used as the outcome of occupational therapy intervention, supporting the broad view defined by AOTA in 1995 (*Position Paper: Broadening the Construct of Independence*).

An attempt has been made to address the comments and requests of students, feedback from instructors and reviewers, and the results of the authors' own intense editing. In large part, this revision arises out of the needs of the readers. The authors are grateful for the opportunity to respond to them in this Fourth Edition.

Module I

THE FOUNDATIONS OF ACTIVITY

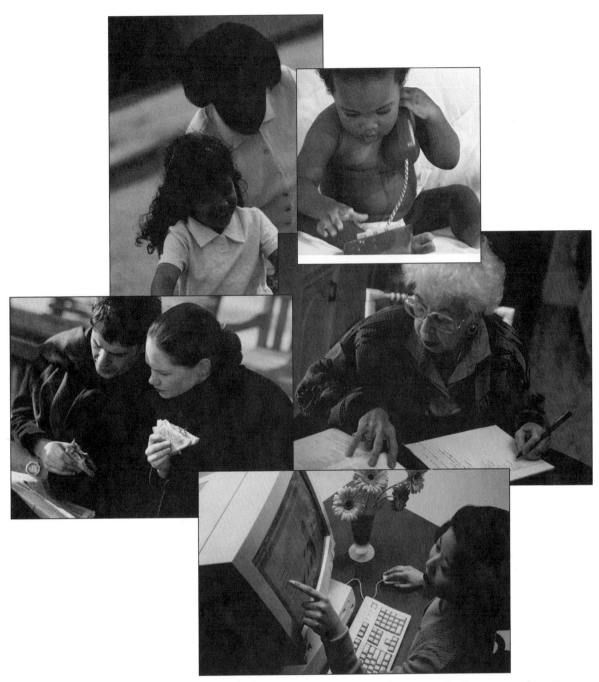

"Occupations are the ordinary and familiar things that people do every day."

Position Paper: Occupation (AOTA, 1995, p. 1015)

Unit One

CONFIRMING REALITY THROUGH OCCUPATION

The human spirit of occupation, developed through eons of time in evolution, unfolding through development, and actualized through daily learning, needs to be nurtured to contribute to the health, quality of life, and survival of persons and society. (Yerxa, 1998)

OBJECTIVES

Upon completion of this unit, the student will be able to:

❖ Understand the vital relationship between occupation and quality of life.

❖ Recognize the importance of using meaningful everyday activities as intervention.

❖ Develop an appreciation of occupation as one of the philosophical roots of occupational therapy.

❖ Consider how the roles of a client impact the goals of therapy.

Historically, occupational therapy began with a focus on what people had to do despite illness or injury. This unit will review the human need for meaningful occupation by briefly examining the writings of selected recipients of the Eleanor Clarke

Slagle Lectureships and other prominent writers of our profession. This examination is but an overview of a portion of our written heritage, and the reader is encouraged to return to these references for further enrichment. The impact of occupation as the basis for treatment will be considered as meaningful intervention and how its use brings credibility to intervention.

As human beings we have an innate need to do. We build, we dismantle, we create, and we repair. We use tools, and if we don't have the appropriate tool at hand, we create one. We use and manipulate all forms of media including space. We occupy our environment and we change it as our needs require. We are born with the curiosity to find out, to try, and to learn through all our avenues of sensing. We invent and then we re-invent. We nurture our progeny, our parents, our family members, and ourselves. We can reach out to offer support to people we don't even know, and we can respond to people who reach out to us. We think, love, laugh, and live. We also pout, argue, and strike out. We have possessions, habits, traditions, and rituals with their significant signs and symbols, as well as laws and mores that provide meaningful attachments to our environment (Fidler & Velde, 1999).

We strive to achieve. We all know persons who have triumphed over seemingly impossible situations because of the innate need to do. At every age, we try, make mistakes, problem solve, and try again. Sometimes when we are overwhelmed with grief and loss, we realize that we cannot continue until we consciously decide to disengage and wait for our well of physical and mental resources to refill. A cup of coffee, a chat with friends or loved ones, a walk in the park, or a vacation can help us regroup. Sometimes we make the decision not to try again. And what are the dynamics of our doing? We are living and consuming. Living is our occupation and we are consuming the experiences of life. We can respond with spirit, optimism, hope, and faith in our environment and ourselves, or be overshadowed by uncertainty, lack of enthusiasm, or in some cases, despair.

"Occupations are the ordinary and familiar things that people do every day" (American Occupational Therapy Association [AOTA], 1995, p. 1015).

In thinking about this definition of occupation, we realize that it has no confining levels of ability or disability. This realization provides avenues of intervention that were unrealized or unavailable when our profession was defined solely by the medical model. Now, with a resurging emphasis on the wholeness of occupation as the basis for practice, clients with or without disability can be served in the context of facility, home, or community.

THE IMPACT OF REALITY ON INTERVENTION

Each client referred to occupational therapy services brings a unique physical and psychosocial status, hopes and fears regarding present and future health, and the influence of significant others. All of these factors are embedded in the content of life experiences and are hinged, one with another. The performance components that require attention are but a piece of the occupational competency puzzle. For example, the impact of cognitive deficits on a child's whole life, not just his or her schoolwork, must be addressed. The occupational therapy practitioner develops an intervention plan to address and integrate all of these factors into the child's goals of meaningful and maximum function.

The reality of occupation for any client is found within the home, the workplace, the educational process, with friends, and in the community. In choosing a real-life setting such as the home as the site of intervention, the practitioner accesses natural resources that can be utilized to enhance the client's occupational performance. By choosing selected elements of reality (or context), the intervention focuses on the center of that client's activity requirements.

Clark (1993) has described the therapeutic value of using true-life experiences as intervention strategies. Research has shown that contrived or non-related activity does not carry over into real-life situations (Thomas, 1996). Fisher (1998) outlines four of the commonly used methods of intervention seen in today's practice: exercise, contrived occupation, therapeutic occupation, and adaptive or compensatory occupation. She characterizes the first two as being therapist-imposed with no meaning or choice for the client. The third method of practice, therapeutic occupation, incorporates the issues of meaning and active participation by the client. The fourth method, adaptive or compensatory occupation, focuses on improving occupational performance through adaptive or remedial measures with no attempt to correct the impairment.

A real-life experience can call into play some of the remnants of former competencies that cannot be easily accessed in a mock-up situation. As an example, an in-home kitchen experience can utilize the client's present assets, environment, and support systems in his or her natural setting. All the background nuances of familiar equipment, weight of utensils, counter height, sink depth, floor texture, ebb and flow of family and pets, fears of new experiences, and pleasures of success are present in therapy experiences couched in a natural setting. On-the-job training, learning to ride a real bus, or taking care of a real baby brings reality to the therapy program. Without these nuances of reality, the competencies noted when the activity is carried out in a clinical kitchen, a mock-up bus, or in diapering a life-size baby doll may not carry over into actual performance.

INSIGHT FROM THE PROFESSIONAL LITERATURE

When life is viewed as occupation, it follows the flow of the thinkers and writers who have offered their research and philosophy on the meaning and value of occupation as the foundation of our profession. Through his research on the persona of Eleanor Clarke Slagle, Bing (1997) offers a delightful look into some of the origins of our developing philosophy that he presents as a scene of a play. The setting is Mrs. Slagle's kitchen in early December 1936. She is sharing some of her own history with three visiting occupational therapists. According to Bing, Mrs. Slagle insisted on using the term "occupational therapy" when speaking of this new profession. She felt that using only the initials "OT" was not informative enough for people to understand this new entity. Bing describes Mrs. Slagle's move to Chicago in 1911 and the beginning of her settlement work at Hull House. There in 1912 she met Dr. Adolph Meyer who was developing his plan for the Henry Phipps Clinic at Johns Hopkins University in Baltimore. This clinic was to house his new concept for treating the mentally ill which he called an "occupational treatment center, a laboratory" (p. 224). He requested permission from Miss Lathrop, the director of Hull House, for Mrs. Slagle to come to Baltimore for 2 years to help develop this new clinic. She was excited to become a part of Dr. Meyer's vision for the care of mentally ill persons that would "provide support, encouragement, guidance, and a firm hand, when necessary, so a person could gain successes with occupations that had curative importance" (p. 224).

Later in the play, she further states her simple belief that occupational therapists:

> *Create situations, using the normal tools of everyday living, to maintain healthy conditions and a situation so that the afflicted individual can effect his own change, his own cure. Change occurs within the patient and we can only encourage it, modify it, and adapt it. (p. 226)*

Friedland (1998) noted that in the early part of the 19th century, both the United States and Canada placed emphasis on the activity and the person. The approach was not on pathology (as with the medical model) "but on the interests and abilities and worked around the pathology to engage the person in occupation" (p. 376). Friedland also noted that the need for rehabilitation services after World Wars I and II, followed by the entry of occupational therapy into the field of pediatrics, required an increased emphasis on personal independence and a decreased focus on occupation in the holistic sense.

Van Deusen (1988) relates Mary Reilly's 1943 conception of the difference between occupational therapy and physical therapy when she wrote: "occupational therapy's purpose is to integrate the fundamental motions elicited by physical therapy into total activities" (p. 146). Today the focus of both professions has changed. Wood (1998) notes that physical therapy's present treatment practice is assuming a closer identification with occupational therapy's traditional goals of functional outcomes in work, self-care, leisure, and recreation (p. 404). She cites the need for occupational therapists to articulate the breadth and depth of our practice and research as "a historical progression of human services dedicated to everyday occupations as instruments of self-actualization, finding one's place in the culture, of realizing effective adaptations and experiencing wellness and health" (p. 408).

Miller (1988) describes how Kielhofner expanded upon the teaching of Reilly to develop the Model of Human Occupation. Clark (1993) and others developed the occupational science project at the University of Southern California. Trombly (1993, 1995), Nelson (1996, 1997), Baum and Law (1997), Gray (1988), and Yerxa (1998), as well as many others, have written in support of the use of occupation as the foundation of our profession. Fisher (1998) describes occupation as a noun of action that enables persons to do and to accomplish, while Christiansen (1999) uses the concept of occupation as the key to identity, goal-setting, and motivation.

In summary, the use of occupation as the main focus for intervention brings the profession back to its roots, providing a solid identity that can be publicly explained and a unifying umbrella that covers all phases of practice. It is also important to recognize that there are those in our profession who view a basis for practice other than occupation (Pelczarski, 2000). Such an open debate provides a healthy venue for research and professional growth.

WHAT MAKES AN OCCUPATION?

There is discussion among the scholars regarding the significance of terms and how many (or few) entities comprise an occupation (AOTA, 1995, 1997). There is discussion in the literature on not only how to use the terms "activity," "task," "occupational performance," "function," and "functional outcomes," but also how to sequence the use of these terms in a way that clearly demonstrates a client's progression toward occupational competence. When does a series of graded activities become an occupation? Can we assume that the occupation of lawn care is made up of a series of blocks of activity (planting, watering, weeding, pest control, and mowing) nested together to form the construct of occupation? How does this construct differ for two clients when one is an elderly gardener with hip degeneration who diligently works in his bed of prized roses, and the other is a professional nursery man who sustained a rotator cuff injury from digging in heavy soil while gardening for a living? Were they not both engaging in their chosen version of the occupation of gardening?

If the answers to these questions are positive, then it can be concluded that each client has a personal set of blocks of activity that must be individually and carefully assembled to form the entity of gardening as occupation for that person. The number, size, and height of the blocks depend upon the purpose for occupational therapy intervention. For the elderly client, the reason is related to the need for leisure skills; for the professional gardener, the intervention is related to the role of work and productivity. The terms "play and leisure," "work and productive activities," and "activities of daily living" are listed as performance areas in *Uniform Terminology* (AOTA, 1994). This document provides the guideline for our professional communication and focuses on the use of a uniform descriptive language of practice. For the purpose of this text, the performance areas of Uniform Terminology will serve as a way of cataloging the occupations that are addressed when using purposeful activity as intervention.

THE SIGNIFICANCE OF ROLES

The first step in developing a meaningful therapy protocol is to develop an occupational history of the client. Trombly (1993) first suggested the practice of assessing from the top-down to gather a sense of the client's life role competence and meaningfulness as a way of clarifying the need for occupational therapy intervention. This differs from a bottom-up approach that first focuses on component deficits that may or may not hinder role function. Fisher (1998) proposed her Occupational Therapy Intervention Process Model as a top-down approach

to evaluation and a framework for developing rationale and implementation of remedial and compensatory intervention.

As the client's life roles prior to the onset of disability are assessed, the following questions must be considered. What are this client's life roles? Are there significant others, family members, or friends that comprise a support system, and what is the status of this system? What is the work history? Are there community involvement or leisure activities? Has the client been successful, adequate, or marginal in these roles? What coping mechanisms, strategies for survival, and spiritual outlooks on life (Peloquin & Christiansen, 1997) are evident?

Evaluation tools have been developed for gathering this information and several current examples follow. Clark (1993) advocates the use of a life history, a narrative of the client's past. Fidler has developed the *Interview Guide: Primary Occupation* (Fidler & Velde, 1999). The *Canadian Occupational Performance Measure* (Law et al., 1994) is a third example. The client's historic occupational roles are as important to the therapy process as the evaluation of the disability. This information helps to develop an understanding of the client's occupational needs and should be an integral part of the initial evaluation. A thorough occupational history provides the compass from which to develop the direction and content of therapy. Costner (1988) states that occupational-centered assessments in pediatrics have not developed as readily as adult assessments due to the lack of a consistent framework. She describes an adaptation of the functional assessment for adults (Trombly, 1993) to "better reflect the unique needs and situations of children" (p. 337).

Through interview and evaluation, the practitioner discerns what the disability means to the client and the caregivers and discovers the human and environmental forces that are relevant to perceived life roles. The practitioner must look beyond the meticulously evaluated pathology to find the resources that can return the client to a meaningful role at home and in the community. When considering the client's status, it is necessary for the practitioner to guard against becoming so caught up in personal professional importance that the client's autonomy as a partner in the therapy process is overshadowed. Developing a mutual partnership leads to the trust and compliance that are necessary for successful therapeutic interaction.

ACTIVITY ANALYSIS AND CLIENT-ACTIVITY CORRELATION

A beginning practitioner learns to analyze any human action in terms of the physical, psychosocial, neurological, and cognitive components as well as the spiritual, developmental, and environmental aspects required to perform that activity. This is the basis for Activity Analysis. Then the value of that activity as treatment is identified and applied to the client's present context of life. This is the Client-Activity Correlation. In the next unit, the student will learn to develop and use each part of the process of activity analysis and its application to therapeutic intervention. The student will learn to select the appropriate tools (meaningful activities that facilitate intervention) and put them at the disposal of the client who will benefit from using them.

DISCUSSION QUESTIONS

1. How has your concept of occupation changed following your reading assignment?

2. How does reality impact occupational intervention?

3. How does the role of the client influence the construct of occupation?

4. Which of your current roles is most meaningful to you, and how does it fit into your present concept of occupation?

5. If your role as a student were to be compromised by a long-term illness, would it change your concept of education as occupation?

REFERENCES

American Occupational Therapy Association. (1994). Uniform terminology for occupational therapy (3rd ed.). *American Journal of Occupational Therapy, 47*(12).

American Occupational Therapy Association. (1995). Position paper: Occupation. *American Journal of Occupational Therapy, 49*, 1015.

American Occupational Therapy Association. (1997). Statement—Fundamental concepts of occupational therapy: occupation, purposeful activity, and function. *American Journal Of Occupational Therapy, 51*, 864-865.

Baum, C. M., & Law, M. (1997). Occupational therapy practice: Focusing on occupational performance. *American Journal of Occupational Therapy, 51*(7).

Bing, R. K. (1997). "And teach agony to sing": An afternoon with Eleanor Clarke Slagle. *American Journal of Occupational Therapy, 51*, 221-225.

Christiansen, C. (1999). Defining lives: Occupation as identity. An essay on competence, coherence, and the creation of meaning. *American Journal of Occupational Therapy, 53*(6).

Clark, F. (1993). Occupation embedded in real life: Occupational science and occupational therapy. *American Journal of Occupational Therapy, 47*, 1067-1078.

Costner, W. (1998). Occupational-centered assessment for children. *American Journal of Occupational Therapy, 52*(5).

Fidler, G. S., & Velde, B. P. (1999). *Activities: Reality and symbol.* Thorofare, NJ: SLACK Incorporated.

Fisher, A. (1998). Uniting practice and theory in an occupational framework. *American Journal of Occupational Therapy, 52*(7).

Friedland, J. (1998). Occupational therapy and rehabilitation: An awkward alliance. *American Journal of Occupational Therapy, 52*(5).

Gray, J. (1988). Putting occupation into practice: Occupation as ends, occupation as means. *American Journal of Occupational Therapy, 52*(5).

Law, M., Baptiste, S., Carswell, A., McColl, M. A., Polatajko, H., & Pollock, N. (1994). *Canadian Occupational Performance Measure* (2nd ed.). Toronto, Ontario: CAOT Publications.

Miller, R., & Keilhofner, G. (1988). In B. R. Miller, K. Stieg, F. M. Ludwig, S. D. Shortridge, & J. VanDeusen. *Six perspectives on theory for the practice of occupational therapy.* Rockville, MD: Aspen.

Nelson, D. L. (1996). Therapeutic occupation: A definition. *American Journal of Occupational Therapy, 50*(10).

Nelson, D. L. (1997). Why the profession of occupational therapy will flourish in the 21st century. *American Journal of Occupational Therapy, 51*(1).

Neufeldt, G. (Ed.). (1997). *Webster's new world college dictionary* (3rd ed.). USA: Macmillan.

Peloquin S., & Christiansen, C. (1997). Occupation, spirituality, and life meaning (special issue). *American Journal Of Occupational Therapy, 51,(3)*.

Pelczarski, M. (2000). Letters to the editor. We cannot hang our hat on occupation alone. *American Journal of Occupational Therapy, 54(1)*.

Thomas, J. (1960). Materials-based, imagery-based, and rote exercise occupational forms: Effect on repetitions, heart rate, duration of performance, and self-perceived rest period in well elderly women. *American Journal of Occupational Therapy, 50,* 783-789.

Trombly, C. (1993). The issue is anticipating the future: Assessment of occupational function. *American Journal of Occupational Therapy, 47(3)*.

Trombly, C. (1995). Occupation: Purposefulness and meaningfulness as therapeutic mechanisms. *American Journal of Occupational Therapy, 49(10)*.

Van Deusen, J. (1988). Mary Reilly. In B. R. J. Miller, K. W. Sieg, F. M. Ludwig, S. D. Shortridge, & J. VanDeusen. *Six perspectives on theory for the practice of occupational therapy* (pp 146). Rockville, MD: Aspen.

Wood, W. (1998). Nationally speaking. Is it jump time for occupational therapy? *American Journal of Occupational Therapy, 52,* 403-409.

Yerxa, E. J. (1998). Health and the human spirit of occupation. *American Journal of Occupational Therapy, 52,* 417.

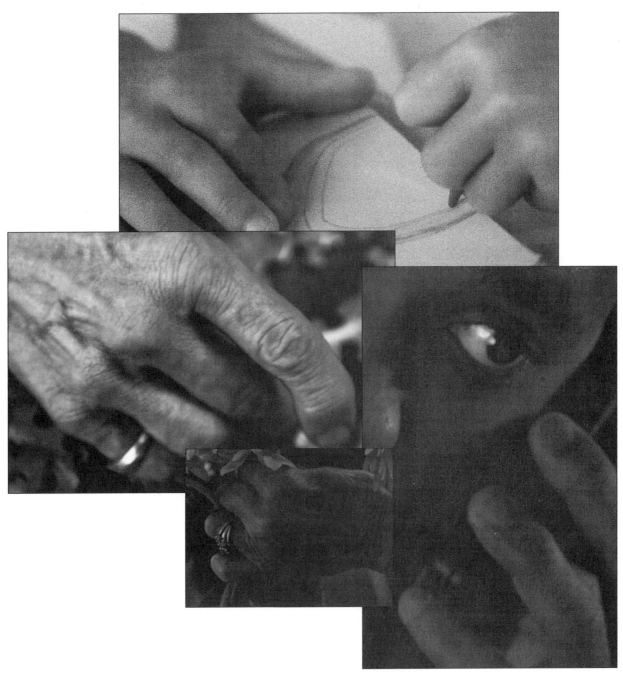

"Man, through the use of his hands, as they are energized by mind and will, can influence the state of his own health."

M. Reilly, 1962

NOTES

NOTES

NOTES

NOTES

Unit Two

EXAMINING THE LEARNING PROCESS OF ACTIVITY ANALYSIS

OBJECTIVES

Upon completion of this unit, the student will be able to:

❖ Value the heritage of occupation and activity intrinsic to the philosophy of occupational therapy.

❖ Distinguish the relationship among the terms "occupation," "task," and "activity."

❖ Describe the connection between health and occupation.

❖ Recognize Uniform Terminology as a language and tool to analyze activity.

❖ Acknowledge the role activity analysis plays in the clinical reasoning process.

❖ Identify the learning approach used in this text.

OUR HERITAGE OF OCCUPATION AND ACTIVITY

A reaffirmation of our heritage has taken hold of the occupational therapy profession. The challenges presented by nontraditional media and other professional philosophies during the 1950s through the 1980s have reawakened the belief in and use of occupation in occupational therapy. Noted thinkers have summoned us to return to our roots dating back to the late 1800s when the value of occupation was proclaimed (Baum, 2000; Fisher, 1998; Reilly, 1962; West, 1984). One of our founders, Adolph Meyer, recognized the value of work and occupation to his neuropsychiatric patients. In October 1921, at the Fifth Annual Meeting of the National Society for the Promotion of Occupational Therapy (now the American Occupational Therapy Association [AOTA]), he stated that "The proper use of time in some helpful and gratifying activity appeared... a fundamental issue in the treatment of any... patient" (p. 1), reflecting his personal commitment to the use of activity in the psychosocial and physical treatment of patients. He described this treatment as the "new scheme." In his words, therapeutic work "was a pleasure in achievement, a real pleasure in the use and activity of one's hands and muscles and a happy appreciation of time" (Meyer, 1922, p. 3). Scattered throughout this historical writing are words like "performance," "balance," "actual doing," "capacities," and "interests" ...words familiar to any contemporary occupational therapist.

Seventy years later, similar meanings of occupation were incorporated into the *Position Paper: Occupation* (AOTA, 1995b): "Occupations are the ordinary and familiar things that people do every day" (p. 1015). This simple-worded definition encapsulates the multidimensional and complex character of occupation. Reminiscent of Meyer's writings, major concepts embedded in the term "occupation" are that it be goal-directed, meaningful to the participant, extend over a period of time, and involve multiple activities (AOTA, 1995b). This multidimensional nature of occupation incorporates performance, contextual, temporal, psychological, social, and spiritual factors. Understanding and applying occupation to intervention programs for our clients becomes a challenge to the novice in occupational therapy.

As noted by Mosey (1986):

> *Purposeful activities cannot be designed for evaluation and intervention without analysis and synthesis. It is this tool that allows the occupational therapist to assess the client's need for intervention and to make a match between the interests and abilities of the client and the activities that will help to meet health needs, prevent dysfunction, maintain function, manage interfering behavior, and bring about growth and change.* (p. 242)

Consequently, an essential skill for any occupational therapist is to become proficient in the dual edge application of analysis and synthesis, i.e., the "process of examining an activity to distinguish its component parts...and the process of combining component parts...to design an activity suitable for evaluation or intervention" (p. 242).

OCCUPATION, PURPOSEFUL ACTIVITY, FUNCTION, AND HEALTH: TERMS AND CONNECTIONS

When the student begins to explore the heritage of our profession, a multitude of definitions and explanations of occupation, purposeful activity, task, and function surface from the literature (Christiansen & Baum, 1997; Moyers, 1999). Over the years, with variations in scope and length, explanations of these terms have emerged. Some terms like "occupation" and "activity" have been used interchangeably (Fidler & Velde, 1999); some theorists have proposed a hierarchy exists within occupation and that tasks and activities are subsets. However, the reflective student will soon realize

that regardless of the period of time or the author, a common thread is present. Occupation used in a purposeful and meaningful way can facilitate the health and well-being of the individual.

To clarify these terms, the Representative Assembly of the AOTA adopted position papers. Beginning with *Purposeful Activity* in 1983, and later revised in 1993, this position paper makes the distinction between occupation and purposeful activity:

> *Occupation refers to active participation in self-maintenance, work, leisure, and play. Purposeful activity refers to goal-directed behaviors or tasks that comprise occupations. An activity is purposeful if the individual is an active voluntary participant and if the activity is directed toward a goal that the individual considers meaningful.* (p. 1081)

In 1995, two additional position papers were created and adopted, one defining occupation and the other function. The *Position Paper: Occupation* (AOTA, 1995b) openly discussed the ambiguity over terms that has occurred over the years in the profession and acknowledged the multidimensional nature of occupation. Though recognizing that additional research and study were needed to fully understand this concept, the position paper did establish occupation as the hallmark of our practice. Prompted by the common use of function by other health care professions, the *Position Paper: Function* (AOTA, 1995a) clarified the role of function in occupational therapy. It declared that function can be used "interchangeably with occupational performance because occupational therapy's domain is the function of the person in his or her occupational roles" (p. 1019). "Function" takes on a comprehensive description of viewing the person performing activities and roles within a prescribed environment.

These terms were brought together in a cohesive manner with the 1999 *Definition of Occupational Therapy Practice for the AOTA Model Practice Act* (Moyers, 1999), adopted in 1999. This document explains that the practice of occupational therapy:

Means the therapeutic use of purposeful and meaningful occupations (goal-directed activities) to evaluate and treat individuals who have a disease or disorder, impairment, activity limitation, or participation restriction that interferes with their ability to function independently in daily life roles and to promote health and wellness. (p. 608)

The "purpose" in purposeful activity is to elicit from the client a calculated response to the activity that addresses the identified intervention goals. Depending upon these goals, the performance of the activity may provide the means to increase strength, encourage social interaction, facilitate self-control, or stimulate cognitive integration. Activities may be graded, structured, or creative; they may effect prevention and adaptation. The key issue is that as the client participates in purposeful and meaningful activity, the activity moves the client toward improved occupational performance.

Ingrained in our history and as defined in the current Practice Act, occupational performance is integral to the promotion of health in the individual. Wilcock (1998) strongly makes this case by arguing two principles. First is that human beings have an "innate need to engage in occupation" (p. 22) not only to satisfy survival needs but also to stimulate and advance themselves. Human evolution is characterized by "ongoing and progressive doings" (p. 22). Second, engagement in occupation is intricately bound to complex health maintenance systems. Without involvement in activity, an imbalance and eventual decline of physical and mental mechanisms results (p. 29). These concepts are central to the philosophy supporting the value of occupational performance.

OCCUPATIONAL PERFORMANCE AND UNIFORM TERMINOLOGY

Ultimately, the outcome of occupational therapy is to enable people to regain health through improved function in the three performance areas of activities of daily living, work and productive activities, and play/leisure activities. Recognizing a need to convey this message in a succinct and universal language, our profession established a standard reporting system entitled Uniform Terminology. The first of these documents was adopted by the AOTA Representative Assembly in 1979. It was later revised and adopted in 1989, and again in 1994 (see Appendix B for the First Edition and Appendix C for the Third Edition). This universal method of language is applicable for client documentation, reimbursement, and research. By having a common language, occupational therapy practitioners can communicate with each other, third-party payers, and other health care practitioners in a manner that greatly reduces communication discrepancies arising from subjective interpretation and unclear terms.

For educational purposes, the occupational performance chart was created to provide a diagrammatical representation of Uniform Terminology. Its intent is to allow the student to both visualize the entire picture of potential intervention scenarios and distinguish each integral part of the system. The three-page representation (Figures 2-1 through 2-3) depicts intervention as a sequential and interactive progression. Performance categories are segmented into workable pieces and then linked together to form potential intervention connections. The first part of the occupational performance chart (see Figure 2-1) provides the three major headings for the succeeding segments. These major headings are:

I. Performance Areas

II. Performance Components

III. Performance Contexts

Figure 2-2, the second part of the occupational performance chart, includes the major categories under each of the three major occupational performance headings. Figure 2-3, the third part of the occupational performance chart, adds all the Uniform Terminology descriptions for each of the above categories. In this way, one segment of the document may be studied and understood before proceeding to the next. In turn, the completed chart provides the student with the potential to develop long- and short-term goals by extracting the performance components to be addressed.

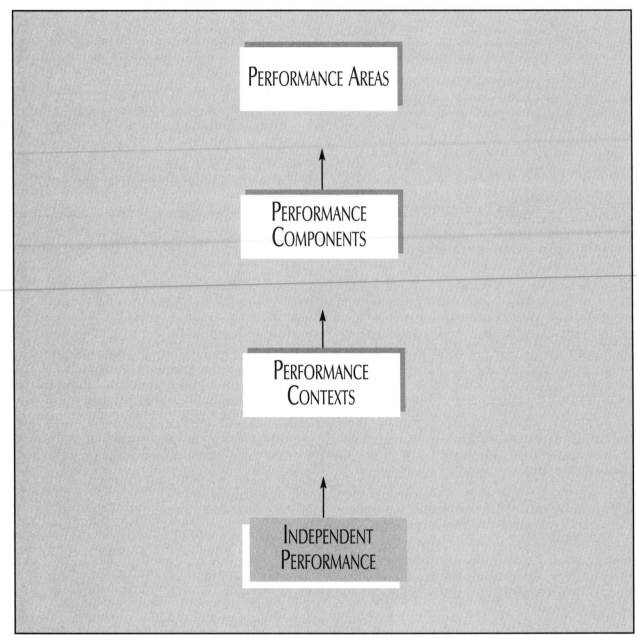

Figure 2-1. Three major headings of Uniform Terminology.

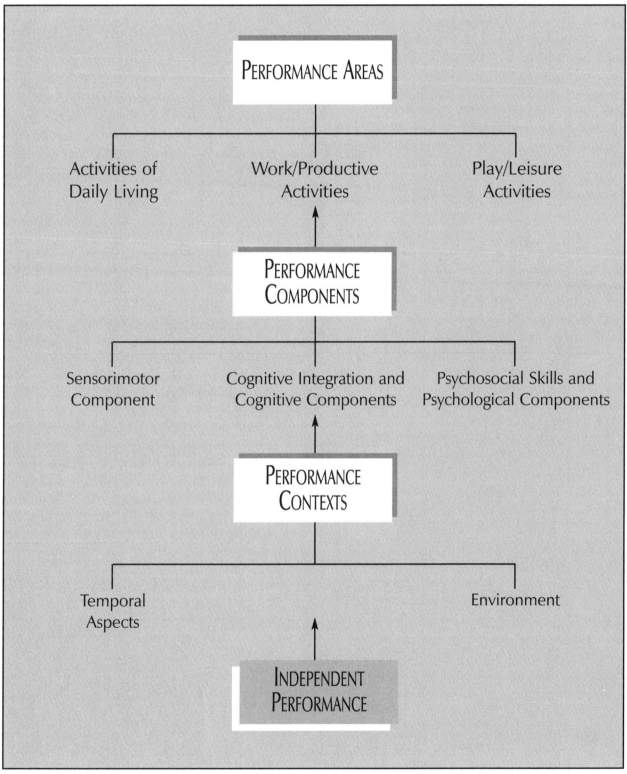

Figure 2-2. Major categories for each of the three major occupational performance headings.

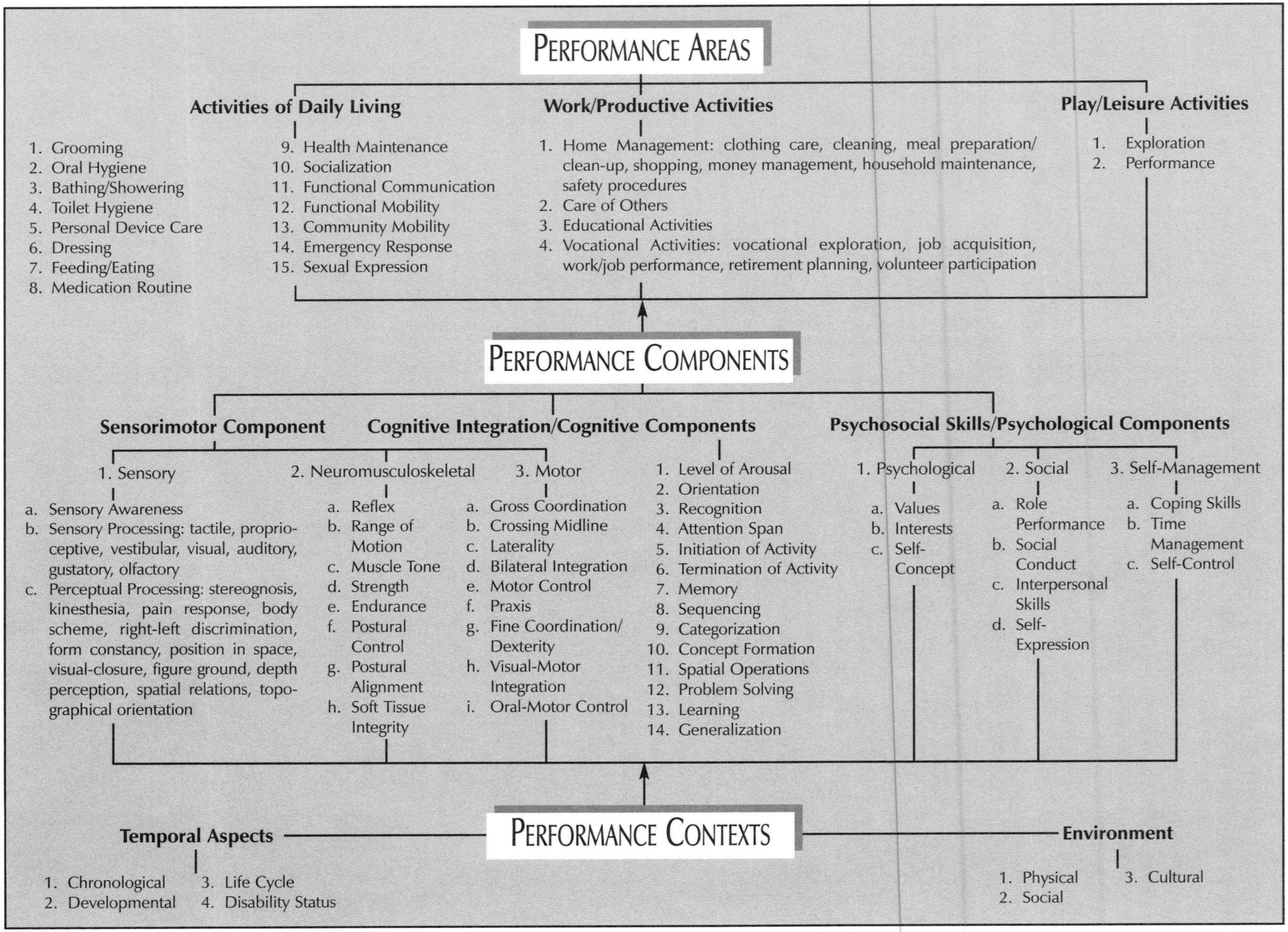

PERFORMANCE AREAS

Activities of Daily Living

1. Grooming
2. Oral Hygiene
3. Bathing/Showering
4. Toilet Hygiene
5. Personal Device Care
6. Dressing
7. Feeding/Eating
8. Medication Routine
9. Health Maintenance
10. Socialization
11. Functional Communication
12. Functional Mobility
13. Community Mobility
14. Emergency Response
15. Sexual Expression

Work/Productive Activities

1. Home Management: clothing care, cleaning, meal preparation/clean-up, shopping, money management, household maintenance, safety procedures
2. Care of Others
3. Educational Activities
4. Vocational Activities: vocational exploration, job acquisition, work/job performance, retirement planning, volunteer participation

Play/Leisure Activities

1. Exploration
2. Performance

PERFORMANCE COMPONENTS

Sensorimotor Component

1. Sensory

a. Sensory Awareness
b. Sensory Processing: tactile, proprioceptive, vestibular, visual, auditory, gustatory, olfactory
c. Perceptual Processing: stereognosis, kinesthesia, pain response, body scheme, right-left discrimination, form constancy, position in space, visual-closure, figure ground, depth perception, spatial relations, topographical orientation

2. Neuromusculoskeletal

a. Reflex
b. Range of Motion
c. Muscle Tone
d. Strength
e. Endurance
f. Postural Control
g. Postural Alignment
h. Soft Tissue Integrity

3. Motor

a. Gross Coordination
b. Crossing Midline
c. Laterality
d. Bilateral Integration
e. Motor Control
f. Praxis
g. Fine Coordination/Dexterity
h. Visual-Motor Integration
i. Oral-Motor Control

Cognitive Integration/Cognitive Components

1. Level of Arousal
2. Orientation
3. Recognition
4. Attention Span
5. Initiation of Activity
6. Termination of Activity
7. Memory
8. Sequencing
9. Categorization
10. Concept Formation
11. Spatial Operations
12. Problem Solving
13. Learning
14. Generalization

Psychosocial Skills/Psychological Components

1. Psychological

a. Values
b. Interests
c. Self-Concept

2. Social

a. Role Performance
b. Social Conduct
c. Interpersonal Skills
d. Self-Expression

3. Self-Management

a. Coping Skills
b. Time Management
c. Self-Control

PERFORMANCE CONTEXTS

Temporal Aspects

1. Chronological
2. Developmental
3. Life Cycle
4. Disability Status

Environment

1. Physical
2. Social
3. Cultural

Figure 2-3. Uniform Terminology descriptions for the categories.

As an example, examine the performance area of activities of daily living which consists of 15 tasks:

1. Grooming

2. Oral Hygiene

3. Bathing/Showering

4. Toilet Hygiene

5. Personal Device Care

6. Dressing

7. Feeding and Eating

8. Medication Routine

9. Health Maintenance

10. Socialization

11. Functional Communication

12. Functional Mobility

13. Community Mobility

14. Emergency Response

15. Sexual Expression

Within the performance area of activities of daily living, the ability to dress may be differentiated into three performance components of sensorimotor, cognitive integration, and psychosocial skills. Then, from each of these performance components, specific skills may be selected as applicable to the client case. For example, sensorimotor considerations may be body scheme, postural control, and praxis; cognitive integration may involve sequencing; and psychosocial skills of self-concept, role performance, and time management could be possibilities.

The third major heading of performance contexts includes temporal aspects and environmental con-

siderations. Any combination of these components could have an impact on the client's engagement in the three performance areas. For example, the client's age, disability status, cultural background, and social surroundings could all have a bearing on the kinds of activities selected for intervention as well as those goals identified as most meaningful to the client.

Returning to the performance area of dressing, two possible scenarios could be:

❖ A 72-year-old woman with a recent stroke and left side hemiparesis whose goal is to independently dress herself and attend her granddaughter's wedding, but presents with left side neglect and weakness and poor self-concept, living alone in subsidized housing.

❖ A 15-year-old female admitted to an adolescent mental health unit for anorexia nervosa who presents with fatigue, negative self-concept, and poor attention to task.

These cases are used to represent how intervention goals may be similar in outcome (i.e., improve dressing skills), yet differ considerably dependent upon the individual's circumstances or context (e.g., age, disability, and socioeconomic status). Uniform Terminology, as configured by the occupational performance chart, is a composite of potential functional outcomes, allowing for individual variation. The purpose of the chart is to provide the student with a diagrammatic portrayal of possible intervention considerations that promote independent performance.

RATIONALE FOR THE ACTIVITY ANALYSIS PROCESS

Since its founding in the early 1900s, occupational therapy has incorporated the process of activity analysis into its basic tools of practice. Creighton (1992) provides a rich chronological description of the inception of activity analysis into the profession. A detailed account is given of writings dating back to 1911, 1920, and 1943 of Gilbreth and Gilbreth, crediting their motion studies in business and industry and their training as mechanical engineers for the advent of "motion analysis" in occupational therapy. Over the years, the scope and depth of activity analysis has taken on many forms (Allen, 1987; Cynkin & Robinson, 1990; Haas, 1922; Licht, 1947; Llorens, 1973). Yet, the core of activity analysis remains the same, that is:

> *…A process that assesses the elements or characteristics of an activity for the purpose of identifying and defining the dimensions of its performance requirements and its social and cultural significance and meanings. It is a process of looking at parts as these relate to defining the whole. (Fidler & Velde, 1999, p. 48)*

Key to intervention is the therapist's ability to analyze an activity and to make that match or synthesize (Mosey, 1986) with the needs and interests of the client. It is a skill that contributes to the therapist's clinical judgment and application of purposeful activity, and in turn, determines the therapeutic effectiveness of the chosen activity. To be successful, activity analysis should include the following features:

❖ Provide the therapist with a thorough understanding of the occupational performance of the activity and the knowledge base for instructing others to perform the activity.

❖ Contribute information regarding equipment, materials, cost, time, space, and staff to perform the activity in the therapy setting.

❖ Generate knowledge to judge for whom, when, where, and under what circumstances the use of the activity is potentially therapeutic.

❖ Detail the therapeutic benefits of the activity when used in intervention.

❖ Supply information useful in documenting an individual's progress in terms of the level of skill required or obtained, difficulties encountered, and reference points for intervention.

❖ Suggest alternative ways and means of performing the activity in an acceptable manner

through adapting or grading the equipment, environment, and/or activity.

❖ Facilitate problem-solving skills in the selection of activities to meet client needs.

❖ Provide a framework from which to formulate intervention goals in the three performance areas for a given client.

❖ Encourage the use of Uniform Terminology to describe, analyze, and document the use of activity in the practice of occupational therapy.

LEARNING APPROACH FOR ACTIVITY ANALYSIS

In a recent article by Yerxa (1998), occupational therapy educational programs are challenged to implement an occupation-centered curriculum that encourages self-directed scholars and generates an autonomous profession. Several concepts suggested for inclusion in this curriculum are grounded in the roots of our profession. One of those identified is activity analysis. The importance of "learning how to assess people's current ability in order to pose a 'just right challenge' …would be stressed" (p. 370).

Taking this charge and implementing it into a meaningful learning experience for future students of occupational therapy presents a weighty challenge. Yet, it is one that is echoed in many camps of the profession. The importance of occupation-based practice and the need for educating students and practicing therapists on the merits of returning to founding values of the profession to become well-versed in the practice of occupational performance is reiterated by Baum (2000). Confirming our own beliefs as educators, the authors felt it important to have a section on the justification of this learning approach to activity analysis included in this Fourth Edition.

It is our belief that the process of learning activity analysis follows a developmental path. The student acquires these skills over time in an evolutionary process. A certain mode of thinking culminates in the ability to see an activity and all its facets, then to match those essential features with the client's needs. In many ways, this process is akin to the clinical reasoning process proposed by Mattingly and Fleming (1994). The assumption is made that clinical reasoning consists of three modes of thinking—procedural, interactive, and conditional. "In a procedural mode of reasoning, therapists search for techniques and procedures that can be brought to bear on the physical problem" (p. 119). "Interactive reasoning [is] used to help the therapists interact with and understand the person better" (p. 120). Conditional reasoning encompasses a greater sophistication and multidimensional art of practice seen most commonly with experienced therapists. In comparison, the analysis and synthesis of an activity could be likened to procedural and interactive reasoning. In that way, they serve as learned strategies that strengthen these modes of thinking.

The intent of this text, then, is to provide the student with a method of developing beginning clinical reasoning skills needed to identify, analyze, grade, and adapt activities used in occupational therapy. In addition, it facilitates the thought processes involved in selecting activities for intervention and further clarifies how purposeful activities can meet specific client needs. To increase personal understanding of the inherent nature and therapeutic benefits of purposeful activity, students are encouraged to examine their own occupational performance and activities as part of this learning process.

The approach to learning activity analysis is multilevel. First, purposeful activity is examined as it is normally performed. This process is called Activity Analysis. Second, specific activities or parts of an activity are matched or correlated with a given client's intervention goals. This process is called Client-Activity Correlation. Five forms are used to teach this multilevel approach and to help the student develop the thought processes required to apply purposeful activity to intervention. Understanding occupational performance and developing skill in using occupation therapeutically are essential features of effective intervention.

The five forms are designed to be used in a sequential manner linking the inherent characteristics of an activity with its therapeutic use. When this way of thinking about activity is applied, the analysis of activity becomes a conscious thought process. The forms are intended to progress the student from a basic understanding of the nature of the activity through the process of breaking it down into its components, and finally matching the therapeutic characteristics of the activity for client intervention. By using the forms, all the major facets of an activity are explored, and the skills needed to engage in it are identified. Students are challenged to problem solve for alternative ways a client can perform an activity when components are impaired or absent. They are also questioned to see how successful occupational performance of an activity contributes to the health of the individual.

The authors believe that intervention outcomes should be observable, measurable, and subject to clear and accurate documentation. In this text, *Uniform Terminology, Third Edition* (1993b), is used as the basis for organizing and documenting the functional outcomes of therapy. This reporting system has been found to be appropriate to document any activity, no matter its complexity, in any intervention plan.

In conclusion, developing the ability to analyze activities is perceived as a multilevel process, one step building on another. By using the forms to examine participation in a number of activities, the student has a wide array of experiences for analysis and synthesis. The final outcome is that the student will feel competent in analyzing and applying activity to treatment.

Specifically, student objectives are to:

❖ Identify the essential features of occupation and purposeful activity and the effect of activity engagement upon an individual.

❖ Describe the occupational performance of an activity in action step sequence.

❖ Analyze an activity in terms of occupational performance areas, components, and contexts.

❖ Identify precautions, contraindications, and acceptable criteria for completion of an activity.

❖ Formulate alternative means of performing an activity in an acceptable manner through adaptation or modification of the task or environment.

❖ Problem-solve the selection of activities that meet the needs of a client receiving occupational therapy.

❖ Propose intervention goals that match the identified needs of the client with the three performance areas.

❖ Apply Uniform Terminology to describe, analyze, and document the use of activities in the practice of occupational therapy.

MULTILEVEL APPROACH TO ACTIVITY ANALYSIS

An occupational therapist examines an activity from at least two different perspectives: as it is normally performed and as it may be potentially performed by a client. Sometimes, "normal" occupational performance can be achieved by the client with little modification or adaptation. Frequently, however, the therapist must restructure an activity to place it within the client's range of abilities or use it to challenge the person to move forward. Along with consideration of these performance components and therapeutic implications, temporal and environmental factors impacting the client's life will also determine the choice of the activities used in intervention.

How, then, does the student organize this myriad of sequential ideas into a manageable structure? Five forms have been developed to provide a template for gathering knowledge of all aspects of an activity and to establish a structure for learning. These forms should be used in the sequence in which they are presented until the student feels competent with them. The forms, then, may be used out of sequence to explore new activities or to approach a different understanding of familiar activities. The activity of "making a phone call" is used to illustrate all five forms. Blank copies of all the forms can be found in Appendix D.

Form 1: Activity Awareness Form

This first form provides an opportunity for an activity to be viewed subconsciously and highlights the student's personal response to a specific activity.

The sensorimotor, cognitive, and psychosocial aspects of the activity are superficially identified.

Form 2: Action Identification Form

The second form provides a more direct approach to the actual performance of the activity. It separates the task into 10 or less sequential steps and also begins the process of observing variations of performing the same activity by several people in a Do-What-How format.

Form 3: Activity Analysis for Expected Performance

The third form provides an intense examination of the occupational performance areas, components, and contexts of the activity. The student is asked to dissect the parts of the activity as it is *normally* performed using the language of Uniform Terminology.

Form 4: Activity Analysis for Therapeutic Intervention

In this fourth form, the student begins to consider what impact deficits or impairment of certain performance components may have upon occupational performance. Activity requirements, intervention implications, and modifications are delineated.

Form 5: Client-Activity Correlation Form

The fifth form provides a structure for the application of an activity as a therapeutic medium in the intervention process. The student is asked to complete a client profile including a description of the specific dysfunction from which long- and short-term goals of therapy are considered. The student suggests an activity that will be used as the intervention medium, describes the preparation and implementation steps, and documents the functional outcomes in the language of Uniform Terminology.

SUMMARY

Occupational therapists need to learn how to use purposeful activity as part of their therapeutic intervention. The multilevel approach used in this text encourages the student to become aware of many different activities and their essential properties. It asks the student to break down activities into steps to identify the specific actions involved in performing them. It requires the student to examine the skills needed to perform those actions, as well as the context in which the activity takes place. Finally, it has the student look at a specific individual's functional deficits and choose an activity that has meaning to the client and that will facilitate occupational performance. Throughout this process, the impact of environment and temporal factors, such as age and disability status, are considered. This approach is applicable to any activity used in occupational therapy and to any intervention setting.

DISCUSSION QUESTIONS

1. What is your understanding of our profession's heritage with occupation and activity?

2. Define "occupation," "activity," and "task." Describe the relationship between these terms.

3. Explain activity analysis in your own words.

4. Identify the major categories of Uniform Terminology. Why does our profession have such a document?

5. What does the phrase "health through activity" mean to an occupational therapist?

REFERENCES

Allen, C. K. (1987). Eleanor Clark Slagle Lecture. Activity: Occupational therapy's treatment method. *American Journal of Occupational Therapy, 41,* 563-575.

American Occupational Therapy Association (1979). *Uniform terminology for reporting occupational therapy services.* Rockville, MD: Author.

American Occupational Therapy Association (1993).

Position paper: Purposeful activity. *American Journal of Occupational Therapy, 47,* 1081-1082.

American Occupational Therapy Association. (1994). Uniform terminology for occupational therapy (3rd ed.). *American Journal of Occupational Therapy, 47*(12).

American Occupational Therapy Association (1995a). Position paper: Function. *American Journal of Occupational Therapy, 49,* 1019-1020.

American Occupational Therapy Association (1995b). Position paper: Occupation. *American Journal of Occupational Therapy, 49,* 1015-1018.

Baum, C. (2000). Reinventing ourselves for the new millennium. *O.T. Practice, January 3,* 12-15.

Christiansen, C., & Baum, C. (1997). *Occupational therapy: Enabling function and well-being* (2nd ed.). Thorofare, NJ: SLACK Incorporated.

Creighton, C. (1992). The origin and evolution of activity analysis. *American Journal of Occupational Therapy, 46,* 45-48.

Cynkin, S., & Robinson, A. M. (1990). *Occupational therapy and activities health: Toward health through activities.* Boston, MA: Little, Brown and Co.

Fidler, G. S., & Velde, B. P. (1999). *Activities: Reality and symbol.* Thorofare, NJ: SLACK Incorporated.

Fisher, A. (1998). Uniting practice and theory in an occupational framework. *American Journal of Occupational Therapy, 52*(7), 509-521.

Haas, L. J. (1922). Crafts adaptable to occupational needs: Their relative importance. *Archives of Occupational Therapy, 1,* 443-445.

Licht, S. (1947). Kinetic analysis of crafts and occupations. *Occupational Therapy and Rehabilitation, 26,* 75-78.

Llorens, L. (1973). Activity analysis for cognitive-perceptual-motor dysfunction. *American Journal of Occupational Therapy, 27,* 453-456.

Mattingly, C., & Fleming, M. H. (1994). *Clinical reasoning: Forms of inquiry in a therapeutic practice.* Philadelphia, PA: F. A. Davis Co.

Meyer. A. (1922). The philosophy of occupational therapy. *Archives of Occupational Therapy, 1,* 1-10.

Mosey, A. C. (1986). *Psychosocial components of occupational therapy.* New York, NY: Raven Press.

Moyers, P. A. (1999). The guide to occupational therapy practice [Special issue]. *American Journal of Occupational Therapy, 53*(3).

Reilly, M. (1962). Eleanor Clark Slagle Lectureship. Occupational therapy can be one of the great ideas of 20th century medicine. *American Journal of Occupational Therapy, 16,* 1-9.

West, W. A. (1984). A reaffirmed philosophy and practice of occupational therapy for the 1980's. *American Journal of Occupational Therapy, 38,* 15-23.

Wilcock, A. A. (1998). *An occupational perspective of health.* Thorofare, NJ: SLACK Incorporated.

Yerxa, E. J. (1998). Occupation: The keystone of a curriculum for a self-defined profession. *American Journal of Occupational Therapy, 52,* 365-372.

NOTES

NOTES

NOTES

Module II

THE DIMENSIONS OF ACTIVITY

Unit Three

FOCUSING ON THE ACTIVITY

OBJECTIVES

Upon completion of this unit, the student will be able to:

❖ Discern the relationship between activity and well-being.

❖ Become aware of hidden aspects of an activity.

❖ Identify action steps in performing an activity.

Activity has a dynamic quality that involves the individual to "actively" participate. The kind of participation varies with the activity, but this energy in doing is present in all activities undertaken. One way to define "activity" is "anything that requires mental processing of data, physical manipulation of objects, or directed movement may be considered an activity" (Trombly & Scott, 1983, p. 243). A more recent definition for the word "activity" is the "productive action required for development, maturation, and use of sensory, motor, social, psychological, and cognitive functions. Activity may be productive without yielding an object" (Christiansen & Baum, 1997, p. 591).

Throughout the lifespan, a person is engaged in activity. A great deal of being alive is just doing things. The decisions concerning what is to be done occupy considerable amounts of time as well. Based on the tasks set before the individual at any moment, activities appear to be selected which hold value and fulfill personal needs. In other words, activities take on significance and are done intentionally. As Adolph Meyer stated, "It is the use that we make of ourselves that gives the ultimate stamp to our every organ" (Meyer, 1922, p. 5).

In a real sense, activities are a vehicle for participating in life, for "being alive." From birth, the newborn engages in activity—-looking, listening, learning. The process of doing becomes more complex as physical and mental abilities develop through childhood and adolescence. By young adulthood, the individual is increasingly involved in the "business" of life: meeting physical needs, attaining personal requirements, and participating as a member in society through school, work, or community responsibilities. Increasing awareness of how to accomplish these tasks in a way to elicit personal satisfaction develops with experience and maturation. Activities are not performed aimlessly, but have a purpose or fulfill one. The individual begins to construct a lifestyle to provide feelings of efficacy, of joy in doing, and in affecting the personal world created (White, 1971, p. 274).

Because of the importance activities hold for humans, several underlying concepts regarding them are summarized as follows.

ASSUMPTIONS ABOUT ACTIVITIES

❖ Activities are primary agents for learning and exploration. Humans affect their world through doing, gaining pleasure and satisfaction through activities.

❖ Activities occur in normal growth and development. Engagement in activities is a part of being human and their intrinsic (built-in) value serves as a vehicle for healing.

❖ Activities have a potential greater than their surface appearance. Multiple areas of function are involved in performing activities, tapping into a variety of body systems including the sensory, neuromotor, and cognitive.

❖ Activities are a means of discovering oneself as well as a way of increasing function (i.e., "being" is embodied in doing). Individuals define much of who they are by what they do and choose to do (Fine, 1980).

Consider how activity is tied to health and well-being. When meaningful activity is not possible, the individual may become incompetent in meeting personal needs and performing developmental tasks. The sense of efficacy declines, and the challenge of life recedes for, in one sense, "to be alive is to have activities worth doing. When there are none, life is weary and worthless" (Reilly, 1977).

Thus a state of inactivity can indicate disability. When an individual loses the skills or ability to interact with the human and/or nonhuman environment, problems in "being, "doing," and "becoming" develop. Movement from one level of achievement and well-being to a lower one may occur. For example, the phrase "I'm not doing anything" has different shades of meaning depending on the person's perspective of wellness. This could signify temporary physical idleness, a mental state of reflection, availability or willingness to engage in activity, an emotional feeling of hopelessness, an actual inability to perform activity, all or none of these ideas.

Health is on a continuum, and the definition of being "sick" has a personal interpretation as well as medical one. When sick with a cold, the number and type of activities one is unable to perform is different than when one is sick with viral pneumonia. Similarly, coping with a broken arm is quite different than compensating for hemiparesis or an upper body amputation. In each of these instances, one is not necessarily "sicker" than another, but the optimum level of performance each person may achieve and the individual's perspective on what defines

health is significant in influencing that person's sense of well-being. In short, the ability to engage in purposeful activity affects the quality of life. "The significance of engagement in activities and the value that such involvement has in sustaining health and a sense of well-being, in shaping quality of one's living and as a therapeutic and rehabilitative endeavor, is universally recognized" (Fidler & Velde, 1999, p. 6). There is a direct relationship between health and occupation (Christiansen & Baum, 1997, p. 14).

UNMASKING THE ACTIVITY: THE ACTIVITY AWARENESS FORM

Objective

Upon completion of the Activity Awareness Form, the student should be able to recognize the hidden facets of an activity as it is performed by a healthy person.

Understanding the inherent qualities of an activity is the beginning step to further analysis and therapeutic application for intervention. To dig beneath the surface appearance of what is happening in an activity can be as elusive as a dog trying to catch his tail. "A person who is involved in purposeful activity directs attention to the goal rather than to the processes required for achievement of the goal" (American Occupational Therapy Association [AOTA], 1993). The underlying side effects of performing activities must be identified by the practitioner to understand the connection between "doing" and "being," between occupation and health.

The intent of the Activity Awareness Form is to tap into the student's stream of consciousness to discover what occurs in the "doing" of an activity. While engaged, the student is unaware of what may be occurring other than what is apparent (e.g., opening a can of soup or sanding wood for a project). Through the use of the Activity Awareness Form, the student is directed to reflect on what is happening behind the scenes, to "catch in the act" the hidden aspects of the activity as it is performed. The focus shifts from the naming of what happened, for example, "making a phone call," to what actually happens during the activity of "making a phone call" (see Form 1-A).

Directions

The student will perform an activity and through use of the form:

❖ Recall the thoughts and feelings spontaneously evoked by the activity. These may include memories, desires, current concerns, or future hopes.

❖ Recognize general requirements of the body to perform the activity.

❖ Express cognitive, physical, or emotional stimulation experienced while doing the activity.

❖ Detect the ongoing effect of an activity after performance is completed.

❖ Identify a personal response to doing the activity.

IDENTIFYING THE COMPONENTS: THE ACTION IDENTIFICATION FORM

Objective

Upon completion, the student should be able to state major steps in performing a familiar activity in one sentence constructions.

As seen above, activities are more than they appear to be. Performing an activity requires the individual to use thinking processes, physical movements, and a variety of skills and functions. The next step in understanding the value of an activity is to distinguish the specific and sequential performance components of an activity from its general appearance. Looking at the major steps required to perform an activity helps to pinpoint the precise "action" taking place.

One method to describe action steps in objective terms is called the Do-What-How style. Based on materials from the Teaching Improvement Project System for Health Care Educators (TIPS), each major step of an activity is described in a brief complete sentence. Steps are recorded sequentially beginning with a verb that indicates what to Do, followed by the specific action with What the per-

son is to perform, and completed by a How phrase to clarify the verb and action (p. 15). Describing in words the actions taking place while doing an activity requires observing what happens on a performance level. Not only are the underlying elements of an activity unmasked, but close attention to the details of the "action" of the activity begins.

The significance of the direction (Do) and the action (What) may be more obvious than the descriptive qualities of the adverb (How). However, the adverb identifies the quality of the action required or observed as illustrated in the following: sit down slowly (a direction) vs. the client appeared to sit down slowly (an observation) (see Form 2-A).

Directions

The student will complete a simple activity and through the use of the form will:

❖ Identify and separate out major specific actions (10 or less) required to perform the activity.

❖ Record the steps in a Do-What-How sentence format.

❖ Observe and record someone else performing the same activity.

DISCUSSION QUESTIONS

1. What activities take up the most time in your life today, and how do these activities differ from those of a year ago? How do your activities differ from your classmate or your instructor?

2. Think of an activity that you derive great pleasure in doing and another activity you are required to do, but in which you take no pleasure. What makes one task enjoyable and the other disliked?

3. Briefly, what action steps comprise one of the above activities? What elements of the activity can you discern are "masked" or hidden beneath the surface appearance of "doing?"

References

American Occupational Therapy Association (1993). Position paper: Purposeful activity. *American Journal of Occupational Therapy, 47,* 1081-1082.

Center for Learning Resources (1979). T.A.S.K. A.C.T. A preinstructional analysis process. Teaching improvement systems for health care educators. Lexington, KY: University of Kentucky.

Christiansen, C., & Baum, C. (1997). *Occupational therapy: Enabling function and well-being.* Thorofare, NJ: SLACK Incorporated.

Fidler, G. S., & Velde, B. P. (1999). *Activities: Reality and symbol.* Thorofare, NJ: SLACK Incorporated.

Fine, S. (1980). *The Richness of activity.* AOTA Video.

Meyer, A. (1922). The philosophy of occupation therapy. *Archives of Occupational Therapy, 1*(1).

Reilly, M. (1977). *Play as exploratory learning.* Beverly Hills, CA: Sage Publications.

Trombly, C. A., & Scott, A. D. (1983). *Occupational therapy for physical dysfunction.* Baltimore, MD: Williams & Wilkins.

White, R. (1971). The urge towards competence. *American Journal of Occupational Therapy, 25.*

Form I

ACTIVITY AWARENESS FORM

Student: <u>Example</u>   Date: _____

Activity: <u>Making a telephone call</u>

Course: _____

Directions: Reflecting on the activity just performed, complete the following sentences with the first words that come to mind.

1. During this activity I was thinking about...

   All the things I need to get done today and hoping the person was home so that I could give her a message she needed before she left home.

2. While doing this activity I felt...

   Relieved when my friend answered the phone and I was able to talk to her.

3. In doing this activity, the parts of my body I remember using were...

   My leg while standing by the phone, my shoulder holding the phone against my ear, writing with my hand while she talked.

4. To do this activity I need to... (mentally, emotionally, physically)

   Remember her phone number, dial accurately, listen for the phone to ring, wait for my friend to respond, relay the information needed, and then replace the receiver.

5. When I do this activity again I will...

   Sit down after dialing the wall phone and have my list in front of me to check off items as I tell them to her.

6. From doing this activity I became aware of...

   How anxious I was to convey the message and complete this job on my list.

Form 2

ACTION IDENTIFICATION FORM

Student: <u>Example</u> _____ Date: _____

Activity: <u>Making a telephone call</u> _____

Course: _____

Directions: Select an activity, and using the Do-What-How style, list the major actions in sequence in 10 steps or less required for you to perform this activity. Repeat the exercise after observing someone else perform the same activity.

OBSERVATION OF SELF

1.   Open phone book deliberately.
2.   Find number accurately.
3.   Lift up receiver firmly.
4.   Listen for dial tone carefully.
5.   Push buttons appropriately.
6.   Listen to other phone ring attentively.
7.   Wait for response eagerly.
8.   Say "hello" clearly.
9.   Conduct and close conversation courteously.
10. Put receiver down securely.

OBSERVATION OF ANOTHER

1.   Find phone number carefully.
2.   Pick up receiver confidently.
3.   Listen for dial tone attentively.
4.   Push numbers correctly.
5.   Listen to ringing patiently.
6.   Talk to person respectfully.
7.   Cease conversation politely.
8.   Hang up receiver firmly.

NOTES

NOTES

NOTES

NOTES

Unit Four

IDENTIFYING THE ACTIVITY

OBJECTIVES

Upon completion of this unit, the student will be able to:

❖ Demonstrate a good working knowledge of Uniform Terminology and apply it to activity analysis.

❖ Analyze an activity as it would be expected to be performed.

ACTIVITY ANALYSIS FOR EXPECTED PERFORMANCE

According to Rogers (1982), to use occupation or purposeful activity effectively for intervention, the occupational therapy practitioner needs to have an in-depth understanding of the health-enhancing nature of occupation. This understanding does not come about through reading or rote memory. It evolves from experiencing "normal" occupational performance and from knowing the therapeutic properties of occupation and the impact that performance deficits have upon occupation.

How, then, does this conceptualization of occupational performance occur? It involves a step-by-step dissection of an activity, whereby the student experiences the activity, uncovers the obvious, analyzes the components of the activity, and discovers its therapeutic characteristics. The intent of the

Activity Analysis Form is to provide the framework upon which this thought process of occupational performance can begin to develop. It is a systematic and comprehensive tool used to analyze a single activity or task.

ACTIVITY ANALYSIS FOR EXPECTED PERFORMANCE: AN OVERVIEW

This portion of the activity analysis is divided into the following two sections.

Section 1: Activity Summary

Nine items are to be identified and described in this section. They include:

❖ The name and brief description of the activity.

❖ Information regarding equipment, supplies, and space/environmental requirements.

❖ The sequence of steps and time required to complete each step.

❖ Precautions and special considerations such as age, educational requirements, and cultural and gender relevance.

❖ Acceptable criteria for a completed activity.

Section 2: Analyzing Occupational Performance Areas, Components, and Contexts

In this section, the dissection of the activity is studied according to three parts: performance areas, performance components, and performance contexts.

Part I: Performance Areas are broad categories that are typically part of everyday life and include activities of daily living, work and productive activities, and play or leisure activities.

Part II: Performance Components are basic human skills that are needed to successfully engage in the performance areas. Three aspects of the self emerge through these components. The sensorimotor components comprise the doing self. The cognitive components are the thinking self, and the psychosocial/psychological components are the feeling and social self (Crepeau, 1986).

Part III: Performance Contexts are factors that influence the client's engagement in the performance areas. They consist of temporal and environmental aspects of the client's world that have an impact upon the performance of the activity.

Objective

Upon completion of the Activity Analysis Form, the student will be able to describe an activity and provide the requirements to perform it as would be expected by a person without deficits.

Directions

To prepare for the completion of the Activity Analysis Form, the student should review the sections "Rationale for the Activity Analysis Process" and "Learning Approach for Activity Analysis" offered in Unit Two. The Activity Analysis Form follows the framework outlined in the *Uniform Terminology for Occupational Therapy, Third Edition* (1993) (see Appendix C). There are two major sections of the Activity Analysis Form, which should be completed according to the following guidelines.

Section 1: Activity Summary requires basic information about the activity. This information should be written in list or narrative form beside each item descriptor.

The student will:

❖ Describe the supplies, equipment, and environmental requirements needed to perform the activity.

❖ Identify the activity sequence and acceptable criteria for completion of the activity.

❖ Indicate the precautions and any other special considerations associated with the performance of the activity.

❖ Provide acceptable criteria for the completed project.

Section 2: Analyzing Occupational Performance Areas, Components, and Contexts is divided into the three performance categories.

The student will:

❖ Describe and analyze the activity using the language of Uniform Terminology.

❖ Examine the performance areas of activities of daily living, work and productive activities, and play or leisure activities; the performance components of sensorimotor, cognitive, and psychosocial; and the performance contexts for temporal and environmental aspects of the activity.

As an example, the student may be asked to address the performance area of activities of daily living, and in particular, the task of dressing. Given that the components of range of motion, fine motor coordination, and right/left discrimination are skills needed to perform that task, the student is asked to analyze an activity like leatherwork to determine its potential for facilitating those skills. The student would provide a brief explanation by each of those components describing how the performance of leatherwork incorporates those skills and could facilitate the task of dressing. If the activity does not directly relate to the performance area, then "n/a" (non-applicable) is written to the right of the item. As the student proceeds through the list of items, think about whether or not the skill is necessary to complete the task as it is normally done (e.g., fine motor coordination is needed in the performance of leatherwork for tooling, lacing, and finishing); if not, write "n/a." To complete the performance contexts, insert the requested information next to the item descriptor (e.g., Developmental—young adulthood; Life cycle—student, mother).

Throughout Sections 1 and 2, it is assumed that the student is performing the activity and the student's own expected responses should be identified, described, and reported. Keep in mind that only the actual performance of the activity described in Section 1: Activity Summary should be analyzed. For instance, if the activity is "leather tooling," then the student assumes that the leather tools and materials are gathered together at the work station and are ready for the activity of tooling. Cutting the leather, applying the design, and preparing the leather are not described as part of the Activity Summary. The scope of the activity described in Section 1 determines the responses asked for in Section 2.

Form 3-A is an example of an activity analysis completed on making a telephone call. Examples of first and third person are provided in the form so that the student can see that an analysis can be addressed from different perspectives. Blank forms are available in Appendix D and on the companion website.

DISCUSSION QUESTIONS

1. Identify the major categories for the Performance Areas, Components, and Contexts. How do you see the relationship between the three?

2. Why are you asked to describe the activity in Section 1 before beginning the analysis?

3. How did you feel as you analyzed an activity? What were you thinking?

4. How do you see activity analysis helping you later as a practitioner?

REFERENCES

American Occupational Therapy Association (1993). *Uniform terminology for occupational therapy* (3rd ed.). Bethesda, MD: Author.

Crepeau, E. L. (1986). *Activity programming for the elderly*. Boston, MA: Little, Brown & Co.

Rogers, J. C. (1982). The spirit of independence: The evolution of a philosophy. *American Journal of Occupational Therapy, 36,* 709-715.

Form 3

ACTIVITY ANALYSIS FOR EXPECTED PERFORMANCE

Student: Example_____Date: _____

Activity: Making a telephone call_____

Course: _____

SECTION 1: ACTIVITY SUMMARY

Directions: Respond to the following in list format.

1. Name of Activity
Making a telephone call from a desk telephone.

2. Brief Description of Activity
The student will prepare to make a telephone call, dial the number, convey a message to a friend, and close conversation.

3. Tools/Equipment (non-expendable), Cost, and Source
Telephone, $10.00, Wal-Mart
Desk and chair, $70.00, Wal-Mart
Address book, $3.00, Wal-Mart

4. Materials/Supplies (expendable), Cost, and Source
Access to phone lines, $20.00, Ameritech
Cost of the call, $1.00, AT&T

5. Space/Environmental Requirements
The activity requires sitting in a chair, behind a desk, in a quiet room at a comfortable temperature.

6. Sequence of Major Steps (in 10 steps or less; specify time required to complete each step)
   1. Sit in chair comfortably   3 sec.
   2. Find phone number in address book accurately   30 sec.
   3. Pick up receiver carefully   2 sec.
   4. Listen for dial tone attentively   2 sec.
   5. Press phone number correctly   10 sec.
   6. Wait for an answer patiently   7 sec.
   7. Talk to person clearly   15 min.
   8. Conclude conversation courteously   5 min.
   9. Put receiver down firmly   2 sec.
                                                        Total time is 21 minutes.

7. Precautions (review "Sequence of Major Steps")
The student should be aware of time constraints and may need to limit phone conversation.

8. Special Considerations (age appropriateness, educational requirements, cultural relevance, gender identification, other)
Student is at an age and has telephone experience to manage phone conversation. Culturally, student needs to be cognizant of time of day and respectful of other person while carrying on conversation.

9. Acceptable Criteria for Completed Project
The purpose of the conversation is accomplished and the phone is put back as initially found.

SECTION 2: ANALYZING OCCUPATIONAL PERFORMANCE AREAS, COMPONENTS, AND CONTEXTS

Part I. Performance Areas

A. Activities of Daily Living

1. Grooming
n/a

2. Oral Hygiene
n/a

3. Bathing/Showering
n/a

4. Toilet Hygiene
n/a

5. Personal Device Care
n/a

6. Dressing
n/a

7. Feeding and Eating
n/a

8. Medication Routine
n/a

9. Health Maintenance
n/a

10. Socialization
Conversation with friend provides social outlet.

11. Functional Communication
The phone call is used to convey information to another person.

12. Functional Mobility
n/a

13. Community Mobility
n/a

14. Emergency Response
n/a

15. Sexual Expression
n/a

B. Work and Productive Activities

1. Home Management

   a. Clothing Care
   n/a

   b. Cleaning
   n/a

   c. Meal Preparation/Cleanup
   n/a

   d. Shopping
   n/a

   e. Money Management
   n/a

   f. Household Maintenance
   n/a

   g. Safety Procedures
   n/a

2. Care of Others
n/a

3. Educational Activities
n/a

4. Vocational Activities

   a. Vocational Exploration
   n/a

   b. Job Acquisition
   n/a

   c. Work or Job Performance
   n/a

   d. Retirement Planning
   n/a

   e. Volunteer Participation
   n/a

C. Play or Leisure Activities

1. Play or Leisure Exploration
n/a

2. Play or Leisure Performance
n/a

Part II. Performance Components

(Both first and second person are used to demonstrate different styles of writing.)

A. Sensorimotor Components

1. Sensory

a. Sensory Awareness

I'm aware of the stimuli around me, such as background noise, close proximity of phone and desk, and the voice of the person with whom I'm talking.

b. Sensory Processing

(1) Tactile

Sense of the receiver in my hand and against my ear, and pressure to push buttons to dial the telephone.

(2) Proprioceptive

Awareness of the placement of the phone in my hand and position of body in the chair and near the desk.

(3) Vestibular

Sense of balance comes into play to maintain sitting position in chair and head control near to phone.

(4) Visual

I can see the phone, the chair, the number in the address book and the numbers on the phone.

(5) Auditory

I hear the dial tone and my friend's voice.

(6) Gustatory

n/a (but I could be drinking a cup of coffee!)

(7) Olfactory

n/a

c. Perceptual Processing

(1) Stereognosis

I am able to identify the receiver in my hand without looking at it.

(2) Kinesthesia

I can sense my arm moving to reach for the phone, dial the numbers, and place the receiver near my ear.

(3) Pain Response

n/a

(4) Body Scheme

Awareness of body parts (e.g., head, arm, fingers) in relation to each other so that accurate movement can occur.

(5) Right-Left Discrimination

The phone is in my left hand as I dial with my right hand.

(6) Form Constancy

The form of the numbers in the address book are the same as the ones I dial on the phone. The phone I'm using now is like the one used at work.

(7) Position in Space
I know where my body is in relation to the desk and phone so that proximity is possible for better access.

(8) Visual-Closure
n/a

(9) Figure Ground
I was able to choose the desired phone number from the printed pages in the address book.

(10) Depth Perception
I can sense the depth of the phone to the table and the numbers on the phone, so I don't reach too short of phone or push too lightly or too hard on touch tone dial numbers.

(11) Spatial Relations
Spatially, I can see where the phone is on the desk in relation to other objects around it (e.g., address book).

(12) Topographical Orientation
I know that I'm in a room where I can access a phone.

2. Neuromusculoskeletal
   a. Reflex
   Nervous system is intact.

   b. Range of Motion
   Sufficient shoulder and elbow flexion and extension to reach for phone and bring to my ear, hand flexion to grasp receiver, and finger manipulation to dial numbers.

   c. Muscle Tone
   Sufficient muscle tension to hold phone to ear.

   d. Strength
   Sufficient strength to overcome gravity to hold receiver to ear and push buttons to dial.

   e. Endurance
   Sufficient tolerance to maintain length of time needed to hold phone and carry on a conversation.

   f. Postural Control
   I can maintain my balance while making the call in a sitting position.

   g. Postural Alignment
   I can sit up straight in the chair while my feet remain on the floor throughout the phone call and conversation.

   h. Soft Tissue Integrity
   The seat is sufficiently comfortable to prevent discomfort and I have the receiver to my ear, maintaining even pressure.

3. Motor
   a. Gross Coordination
   Some large muscle movement in trunk, shoulder, and elbow for reaching motion is required.

   b. Crossing the Midline
   This motion occurs in picking up receiver, dialing the number, and bringing receiver to ear.

c. Laterality
I use my dominant hand to dial the number.

d. Bilateral Integration
One hand holds the receiver to the ear while the other hand dials the number. I use both hands at the same time to flip through address book to find the correct number while holding the book.

e. Motor Control
Muscles allow arms and hands to move in a smooth way to complete the task of making the call.

f. Praxis
Motor movements occur in an organized sequence in order to make and complete the phone call.

g. Fine Coordination/Dexterity
This is needed for me to turn pages in address book, lift receiver off phone, and dial the numbers.

h. Visual-Motor Integration
I look at the number in the address book and then dial it.

i. Oral-Motor Control
I use the muscles of my mouth and throat to produce sounds and form them into words.

B. Cognitive Integration and Cognitive Components
1. Level of Arousal
I'm alert enough to find the number in the address book and complete the task of making the phone call.

2. Orientation
I know who and where I am so that a phone call can be made. I am also aware of the time of day and whether or not it is an appropriate time to make the call.

3. Recognition
I can recognize the task as one I have done before and with which I am familiar, as well as the voice of the person whom I'm calling.

4. Attention Span
Adequate attention is needed to complete the call.

5. Initiation of Activity
I am capable and knowledgeable enough to sit at the desk, open the address book, and dial the number to begin the task of conversation with friend.

6. Termination of Activity
I am capable of ending the conversation in a timely manner.

7. Memory
I can recall the purpose and procedure of making a call (e.g., the sequence of steps needed to complete the task).

8. Sequencing
I can perform all the steps necessary to make the call in correct order.

9. Categorization
I know to use an alphabetical order of names in the address book to find the correct name and number.

10. Concept Formation
This is needed to organize incoming and outgoing information so as to convey my thoughts during the conversation.

11. Spatial Operations
I can manipulate the receiver from the phone set to my ear and down again.

12. Problem Solving
I recognize the need to make a phone call to my friend, plan what I will say, note that I could email her or just wait, but decide to make the call, proceed with the call, and follow-up the conversation with the outcome we decided upon.

13. Learning
This is a skill I already know how to do, so no new learning took place.

14. Generalization
I have made calls before and have that as a reference to successfully compete the task.

C. Psychosocial Skills and Psychological Components
1. Psychological
   a. Values
   I value my friendship and believe that my friend will feel the same way, as we have talked together on numerous occasions.

   b. Interests
   My friend and I share mutual interests so that our conversation will reflect those ideas and feelings.

   c. Self-Concept
   I feel positive about calling my friend and having a conversation with her, as I know that she too will feel good that I have called her.

2. Social
   a. Role Performance
   I play the role of friend to the person whom I am calling.

   b. Social Conduct
   Certain telephone etiquette is needed to carry on a phone conversation.

   c. Interpersonal Skills
   I interact with my friend using verbal skills and active listening.

   d. Self-Expression
   I can change or control my speech and thoughts in order to express myself to my friend.

3. Self-Management
   a. Coping Skills
   I need to be able to handle any conversation topic that may be presented so as to carry on a civil discussion for the duration of the phone call.

   b. Time Management
   Monitoring time spent on the phone is required.

   c. Self-Control
   I need to maintain control over my behavior in response to my friend's feedback while we are conversing.

Part III. Performance Contexts

A. Temporal Aspects

1. Chronological
I am 25 years old.

2. Developmental
Young adulthood, and able to manage such tasks as a phone call.

3. Life Cycle
Student in college.

4. Disability Status
n/a

B. Environmental Aspects

1. Physical
All the necessary non-human objects are present for me to conduct a phone conversation (e.g., desk, chair, phone, address book).

2. Social
The phone call serves as an available social outlet with my friend.

3. Cultural
The custom of making a phone call and meeting the behavior standards of such an activity are part of my environmental context.

NOTES

NOTES

NOTES

NOTES

Module III

THE THERAPEUTIC UTILIZATION OF ACTIVITY

Unit Five

DEVELOPING THE ACTIVITY

Thus, the unique contribution of occupational therapy is to maximize the fit between what it is the individual wants and needs to do and his or her capability to do it. (Christiansen & Baum, 1997, p. 40)

OBJECTIVES

Upon completion of this unit, the student will be able to:

❖ Define the terms "grading" and "adapting" as applied in occupational therapy intervention.

❖ Explain how grading or adapting activities can contribute to improving the client's performance.

❖ Give examples of a graded activity in each of the occupational performance areas.

❖ Give examples of adaptations in each of the occupational performance areas.

❖ Recognize specialty areas in service delivery related to grading and adapting activities.

With a thorough understanding of how to perform an activity, the student can begin to see ways in which the activity can be graded or adapted to meet specific client needs. Like analysis, there is no one way to grade or adapt activities. Both gradation and adaptation are used in the process of intervention to help a client change performance. The practitioner determines the intrinsic values within an activity through analysis and then may grade or adapt the activity to develop its potential value to a specific client (Trombly & Scott, 1977, p. 243). In this unit, several approaches to grading and adapting activities will be shown.

"An occupational therapy practitioner grades or adapts a chosen activity for an individual to promote successful performance or elicit a particular response" (American Occupational Therapy Association [AOTA], 1993).

For the purposes of this unit, grading will refer to changing the complexity of what is to be performed, and adapting will refer to modifying or substituting objects used in performing the activity.

GRADING

Grading activities are a part of daily life. Making a list of errands to do and checking them off as they are completed is a graded activity. Separating laundry into piles of dark- and light-colored clothes before placing them in the washing machine is another example.

Grading activities challenge the patient's ability by progressively changing the process, tools, materials, or environment of a given activity to gradually increase or decrease performance demands. These incremental modifications are made in response to the individual's dynamic changes and provide opportunities for gradual development of skill and related therapeutic benefits. (AOTA, 1993)

Grading means to arrange or position in a scale of size, quality, or intensity. Grading can be compared to measuring how much of a specific task is performed. Most students experience "being graded" in school, in other words, how they measure up against a given standard. Grading involves setting a goal and then backing off to see how to complete it: the number of steps to be taken, the amount of time to be given each one, and the details required to perform them. In one sense, it is reversing the analysis of an activity. Performing the activity is the goal. The challenge is how the client will do the activity given specific strengths and limitations. The method used to reach that goal must be chosen by the therapist using professional experience and expertise to determine the appropriate means. Grading the activity is comparable to setting the stage for the client to succeed in performing it.

Some common examples of grading include:

❖ Breaking a lengthy activity into smaller units with given endpoints instead of tackling the entire job, such as threading only 1 inch at a time of a weaving pattern that may be several inches long.

❖ Organizing items logically and in location according to priority use instead of having them in the general work area, such as placing writing utensils and paper on the desk on the dominant hand side.

❖ Changing the amount of energy needed by using lighter weight materials or tools to complete a project, such as working with softwoods (pine or poplar) instead of hardwoods in making a bookcase or using a power saw instead of a handsaw for cutting the wood.

❖ Increasing or decreasing the number of repetitions of an activity, such as walking a longer distance to improve endurance or doing less keyboard work to rest wrist extensor.

Another way of looking at grading is comparing the process to normal growth and development. As a toddler, it is normal to play with a telephone (real or replica) such as turning the dial or pushing buttons, holding the receiver, talking to an imaginary friend, and placing the telephone back in the cradle. As a child grows, the mechanical and proper use of a telephone takes on importance, including skills such as obtaining correct numbers, understanding the significance of these numbers, and listening as well as replying. Later, additional skills are added: to look up specific numbers by alphabetical order, to make and receive calls, respond courteously, limit phone conversations in time or subject, handle phone options such as call forwarding, and perform long distance or credit card calls. A toddler would not be expected to perform the activity of making a phone call on the same level as an adult. By grading the activity to what is appropriate to the individual's ability, the occupational therapy practitioner provides the setting, opportunity, and means for the individual to adapt and master the task.

For example, telephoning a beauty parlor to make an appointment is the purposeful activity chosen for a client experiencing mild confusion and problem-solving skills following a seizure. The therapist may grade the activity on a continuum from one extreme to the other based on the client's needs and progress as follows:

❖ All items assembled in one area for client use, gradually changing to the client locating and retrieving all items needed to perform activity.

❖ No time constraint placed on client to complete activity, gradually changing to a set amount of time in which to perform activity.

❖ Working without distraction in a quiet setting, gradually changing to working with background noise and frequent interruptions.

❖ Providing verbal cueing and a written sequence of steps, gradually changing to self-initiated activity.

❖ Role modeling the phone call, gradually changing to spontaneous independent performance.

Activity grading is used by the therapist to help a client improve performance level. Most activities involve overlapping use of multiple skills. In the above example of making a phone call, an activity analysis provides the information that sensorimotor, neuromuscular, cognitive, and psychosocial components are all involved when performing this activity. The task characteristics are also identified and give important information for use in grading the activity. Through gradual changes of the temporal aspects and environmental needs to perform the activity, the client is provided the means for gradual improvement in occupational performance. "As a general rule, an activity should be graded up when the patient is able to accomplish the task and further progress is desired, or graded down when the patient is having difficulty with performance" (Levine & Brayley, 1991, p. 610).

Consider a graded exercise and activity program in a cardiac rehabilitation unit of a hospital. The first intervention session may involve passive range of motion to all extremities of the client and teaching proper breathing techniques. The client may be allowed to perform oral hygiene and feed self with the bed elevated at a 45-degree angle and with arms supported, but is dependent on nursing for bathing and dressing. By the fourth session, the client may have progressed to performing active range of motion to all extremities with the bed in a 45-degree angle. The client may now be able to wash the front of the torso and use a bedside commode. By session eight, the client may be standing with 1- to 2-pound weights to perform range of motion exercises, bathe in a tub with assist getting in and out, and begin independent dressing activities. The gradual increase in occupational performance can be well-documented and illustrates the use of grading.

Knowing the client's occupational history is an important resource for determining how to grade the activity. The individual's anxieties, interest level, and expectations regarding therapy help the practitioner determine where and how to focus on improving performance. In the above example, the activity of making a phone call to set up an appointment may range from being the infrequent task of a homemaker to the major job component of an executive assistant. The significance of performing specific components of this activity used in a variety of activities versus performing this one activity successfully as part of the person's occupational needs is an important distinction to be made.

Another aspect of grading is looking at where occupational therapy intervention should begin. There are many types of standardized forms to "grade" the client's ability to function during an evaluation. Observing clients perform a functional task such as oral hygiene, feeding, dressing, or homemaking can pinpoint problems in attention, memory, initiation, safety and judgment, problem solving, visual tracking, body awareness, and/or motor planning. Through grading their performance, the practitioner identifies more precisely the specific disability. The intervention can begin at a point where the client successfully performs with subsequent sessions gradually increasing the demands on the client's occupational performance.

Every activity used in occupational therapy intervention should be gradable. With that prerequisite, every activity used has the potential for documenting the client's progress.

ADAPTATION

A background in the historical and conceptual use of the term "adaptation" in occupational therapy is beyond the scope of this book, but is an important part of the student's education. A list of references is given at the end of this unit as a starting point for learning more. In one sense, the real goal of all occupational therapy is to facilitate the client's adaptive responses to promote health and well-being.

What is an adaptation? Simply put, something that makes doing some activity easier. Technically, an adaptation is a change in structure, function, or form that provides a better adjustment to the environment in which people live. For the purposes of this textbook, the term "adaptation" is being used as defined in the statement below.

Therapeutic adaptations refer to the design and/or restructuring of the physical environment to assist self-care, work and play/leisure performance. This includes selecting, obtaining, fitting and fabricating equipment, and instructing the client, family and/or staff in proper use and care of equipment. It also includes minor repair and modification for correct fit, position, or use. (AOTA, 1979)

Adaptations surround us daily. As humans, we are constantly looking for ways to perform activities competently, effectively, and efficiently. Some common examples of adaptations are:

❖ Applying Velcro to serve as a fastener on the flap of a purse.

❖ Color coding files of information for quick retrieval.

❖ Recording foreign language phrases on a cassette to play/pause/repeat as needed.

❖ Marking the grain of the fabric with a safety pin to lay out a dress pattern.

❖ Wearing a Walkman to weed out unpleasant stimuli while working.

❖ Putting different textured surfaces onto individual keys to aid in finding the correct one.

Adaptation may require changing the tool or technique used to perform an activity. The therapist must judge whether or not to use a device to substitute for a specific performance component designed to function in place of the client's ability. Using a stationary cutting board to substitute for bilateral function in slicing vegetables or installing a grab bar in a bathroom to facilitate transfers are examples of adaptations.

Adaptations do not change the outcome of an activity, but the means of accomplishing the activity is purposefully altered to make it within reach of the client's ability. Looking up a phone number and dialing it may be a difficult task for the client experiencing hemiparesis, loss of memory from a head injury, or severe depression. Adaptations may include setting up a Rolodex to replace a phone book, learning to use a redial feature on a phone console, or plugging a headset into the receiver instead of handling the traditional one.

In some instances, the therapist may decide not to adapt the activity used in intervention. The client may be working to reach the same level of function before disability occurred including doing the activity as it was "normally" performed prior to dysfunction. For example, a woman suffering from a stroke may benefit from using a plate guard while eating, but be motivated to learn how to perform without it. The client may also resist or deny the need to have adaptations until the need is clearly demonstrated. For example, a person experiencing a double below the knee amputation may feel learning to wear prosthetics is discouraging and a bother until the desire to be independent in a public restroom provides the meaningful incentive for using them. The client may also have a preference to perform activities in a specific way despite the timeliness or expenditure of physical energy involved. The purpose and meaning attached to the way in which the activity is accomplished may be more important than making the task easier. For example, a man with multiple sclerosis may choose to use leg braces rather than a wheelchair to walk down the aisle at his daughter's wedding. The therapist must know when to subordinate personal preferences to the client's desires, yet not jeopardize the welfare and safety of the client. Again, the client's occupational history is an important component of knowing when an adaptation is needed and what is an appropriate one to use.

Occupational therapy practitioners are increasingly involved in delivering services in specialty areas of practice. Two of these are mentioned here because of their specific use of skills in adapting and grading activities. *Ergonomics* is a field of study using applied science to specifically adapt equipment and the surrounding work environment to maximize human productivity. Adapting working conditions to suit the worker includes the physical space, lighting, and sensory input, as well as tools and equipment.

Assistive technology is formally defined as "any item, piece of equipment, or product system, whether acquired commercially or off the shelf, modified, or customized, that is used to increase, maintain, or improve functional capability of individuals with disabilities" (Public Law 100-407, Technology-Related Assistance for Individuals with Disabilities Act of 1988). The use and development of technology or applied science has exploded in the past half century to affect people around the world in a myriad of ways. In all its varied shapes and forms, from basic devices such as long-handled reachers, to complex environmental control units, to general information technologies such as the Internet, assistive technology is within the scope of occupational therapy service delivery when applied to enhance an individual's performance. Technology can be an important tool to the practitioner when used appropriately to enhance an individual's occupational performance. Like prosthetics and orthotics, assistive technology is one of the categories of therapeutic adaptations.

The rapid pace with which changes and new developments are taking place in both ergonomics and assistive technology has created a demand for personnel with the proper qualifications to fill this need. Occupational therapists are well-suited to work in both of these fields because of their skill in adapting activities or the setting to match the individual's needs.

Three further points should be mentioned regarding grading and adaptation. First, it is important not to contrive inappropriate activities as a means of grading or adapting them to improve client performance—for example, having the client roll putty into pea-size balls to simulate eating them with a fork rather than dining with actual food and utensils in the cafeteria, or fastening a weight to a hanger to improve upper extremity strength and endurance rather than hanging a variety of garments of different weights. The activity should be meaningful as well as purposeful while matching goals of intervention. Whenever possible, avoid substituting for the actual situation in which the client will perform and provide realistic gradations.

Second, the practitioner often must choose between fabricating an adaptation using clinic time and materials or buying a commercial product to do the same job. It may be more cost-effective to purchase a similar product and modify it to fit when received. On the other hand, a manufactured item may not be available or not have the capability of being customized for the individual and require the therapist to pursue other solutions. Similarly, in some instances it may be more efficient to have the client perform a commercially produced activity than to devise one to facilitate the desired response. Liability of the product used or the practitioner's own occupational readiness to perform certain physical modalities are other considerations. Again, knowledge, experience, and the individual client's response to the activity will enter into the decision of how the therapist will proceed with intervention.

Third, the practitioner must personally be able to grade and adapt professional performance. In other words, the therapist grades and adapts not only activities used in intervention, but also personal behavior to meet the client's needs. The therapist must adjust and "fit" modalities given multiple variables: the client's health status, time restraints, resources available, the acceptable practice standards, physician approval, and other therapy requirements to name a few. In a sense, the practitioner is the master role model of demonstrating adaptive behaviors and facilitating the adaptive response in the client's occupational performance.

DISCUSSION QUESTIONS

1. How have you changed in your ability to perform successfully in school since kindergarten? High school? College? How has "grading" influenced this ability?

2. What are some common adaptations you use in your own life? In what way do they make the activity easier to perform?

3. When you are ill, in what ways do you grade the activities you are able to perform?

4. Why are occupational therapy practitioners well-qualified to contribute in the fields of ergonomics and assistive technology?

References

American Occupational Therapy Association (1979). *Uniform terminology for reporting occupational therapy services*. Rockville, MD: Author.

American Occupational Therapy Association (1993). Position paper: Purposeful activity. *American Journal of Occupational Therapy, 47*, 1081-1082.

Christiansen, C., & Baum, C. (1997). *Occupational therapy: Enabling function and well-being* (2nd ed.). Thorofare, NJ: SLACK Incorporated.

Levine, R. E., & Brayley, C. R. (1991). Occupation as a therapeutic medium: A contextual approach to performance interaction. In C. Christiansen & C. Baum (Eds.). *Occupational therapy: Overcoming human performance deficits* (pp. 591-631). Thorofare, NJ: SLACK Incorporated.

Public Law 100-407, Technology-Related Assistance for Individuals with Disabilities Act of 1988.

Trombly, C. A., & Scott, A. D. (1977). *Occupational therapy for physical dysfunction*. Baltimore, MD: Williams & Wilkins.

NOTES

NOTES

NOTES

NOTES

Unit Six

UTILIZING THE ACTIVITY

OBJECTIVES

Upon completion of this unit, the student will be able to:

❖ Describe the therapeutic qualities of the activity.

❖ Identify possible gradation and adaptation strategies for the activity.

❖ Begin to formulate intervention outcomes for specific population-based groups.

ACTIVITY ANALYSIS FOR THERAPEUTIC INTERVENTION

This form takes the student one step beyond activity analysis. The intent is to have the student begin to think like a practitioner (as if the activity will be used with a client). The potential for the activity to be purposeful and meaningful for intervention is explored. Here is where consideration of the activity as a therapeutic modality is addressed. To assist the student in translating the performance areas, components, and contexts of the activity into a therapeutic mode of thought, this form is divided into three sections. Each section represents a hierarchy of levels demanding the student to think

more intensely about the client status in comparison to the expected task performance.

Section 1: Activity Description

The student provides a brief description of the activity being analyzed for therapeutic value and identifies the major steps in performing the activity. Initially in the learning phase of activity analysis, when an activity has been analyzed using the first Activity Analysis Form, this section does not need to be repeated for that activity. However, as the student becomes more competent in this thought process, this section should be completed if the first form was not done. This will be especially true as new activities are added to the student's repertoire of experiences.

Section 2: Therapeutic Qualities

In this section, characteristics of the activity that have therapeutic potential are identified in terms of energy and activity patterns elicited by its performance. For example, in performing leather tooling, a moderate work energy pattern is typically used as demonstrated through respiratory and tolerance demands upon the person. Activity patterns may exhibit varied characteristics (e.g., leather tooling is somewhat methodical and repetitive, yet can be expressive in design).

Section 3: Therapeutic Application

This section allows the student to consider for whom and in what way occupational performance can be enhanced by engaging in the activity. At this point, the student now applies the concepts of gradation and adaptation learned in Unit Five. Particular attention is given to ways in which the activity can be adapted to a client's needs as well as how preventative measures may be implemented to facilitate optimal occupational performance. Finally, the student is asked to consider how the activity may play a part in the balance of the performance areas to enhance the health of the client.

Objective

Upon completion of the form, Activity Analysis for Therapeutic Intervention, the student will be able to address the therapeutic implications of any given activity.

Directions

❖ Describe characteristics of the activity including energy and activity patterns.

❖ Formulate possible intervention outcomes that could be derived from engaging in the activity.

❖ Explain gradation and adaptation possibilities.

❖ Specify therapeutic modifications which may be made to the activity, with the client, and/or to the environment to achieve identified goals.

Before completing this form, the student should review *Uniform Terminology for Occupational Therapy, First Edition* (1979), for definitions of terms used in the Therapeutic Modifications portion (see Appendix B).

Form 4 is an example of making a telephone call.

DISCUSSION QUESTIONS

1. What have you learned about therapeutic implications that is most interesting to you? Most challenging?

2. What do you see as the next step in learning more about activity analysis?

REFERENCE

American Occupational Therapy Association (1979). *Uniform terminology for reporting occupational therapy services.* Rockville, MD: Author.

Form 4

ACTIVITY ANALYSIS FOR THERAPEUTIC INTERVENTION

Student: <u>Example</u>   Date: _____

Activity: <u>Making a telephone call</u>

Course: _____

SECTION 1: ACTIVITY DESCRIPTION

A. Provide a Brief Description of Activity
The student will prepare to make a telephone call, dial the number, convey a message to a friend, and close conversation.

B. Identify Major Steps
1. *Sit in chair comfortably.*
2. *Find phone number in address book accurately.*
3. *Pick up receiver carefully.*
4. *Listen for dial tone attentively.*
5. *Press phone number correctly.*
6. *Wait for an answer patiently.*
7. *Talk to person clearly.*
8. *Conclude conversation courteously.*
9. *Put receiver down firmly.*

SECTION 2: THERAPEUTIC QUALITIES

A. Energy Patterns—Describe the required energy level in terms of light, moderate, or heavy work patterns and provide an explanation for the level specified.

Minimal to moderate work pattern is needed to complete the activity. The person needs to focus and organize self while preparing and completing it. Cognitive awareness and required physical actions to perform the activity demand some mental and physical exertion, but typically this is considered a sedentary activity.

B. Activity Patterns—Indicate the patterns of the activity expected for successful completion of the activity.

1. Structural/Methodical/Orderly
Steps of activity provide structure and order to perform the activity (e.g., have address book available to find number, pick up receiver, and use phone to dial number).

2. Repetitive
n/a

3. Expressive/Creative/Projective
Verbal expression is utilized during the conversation to exchange thoughts and ideas.

4. Tactile
    a. Contact with Others (e.g., hands-on, stand by assist)
    This activity does not require physical contact with others.

    b. Materials (e.g., pliable, sensual)
    Hands and fingers are touching the cover and pages of address book; hand, fingers, face, and ear are on receiver; fingers touch the dial; and body sits on chair. Materials are mostly of a solid surface except for pages of book.

    c. Equipment (e.g., size, manageability, shape)
    Telephone is of the right size and shape for effectively managing the call; desk and chair are appropriate for activity.

SECTION 3: THERAPEUTIC APPLICATION

A. Population—Discuss for whom and in what way increased occupational performance can be derived from the use of this activity. Consider the sensorimotor, cognitive, and psychosocial aspects. Identify any contraindications.

This activity falls in the performance areas of functional communication and socialization. In the sensorimotor realm, it promotes fine motor coordination/dexterity, bilateral integration, auditory sense, and praxis.

Cognitively, it facilitates several components, including attention, memory, sequencing, planning, and implementing an activity. Psychosocially, it may reinforce values and interests, enhance self-concept, social conduct, and interpersonal skills, and requires time management.

No apparent contraindications, unless social behaviors are severely dysfunctional or there is a possibility the phone could be used abusively.

Population-based groups for which this activity could have applicability are: deficits in fine motor coordination/dexterity and grasp as seen with muscle weakness or paralysis; cognitive deficits in sequencing, attention to the activity, problem-solving; and psychosocial problems of social conduct and interpersonal skills.

B. Gradation—Describe ways to grade this activity in terms of:

1. Activity Sequence, Duration, and/or the Activity Procedures

The activity sequence could be graded from supervision of practitioner to independent performance of client (e.g., instructions could be written or in picture format, the activity could be broken into smaller parts for easier manageability, or client could be asked to initiate and implement activity on own).

Duration of call could be shortened or lengthened, depending on client's capabilities or purpose of call.

Activity procedure could be altered by using different types of communication (e.g., email or cellular phone). It could be done with a friend or stranger. Purpose of call could vary from utilitarian as a request for information to more social.

2. Working Position of the Individual

The client could be asked to stand by a wall phone, sit in another type of chair, or make call from a bed, and/or asked to retrieve materials for the activity, depending upon the endurance of client.

3. Tools
   a. Position
   The phone and address book can be placed in various planes depending upon the needs of the client for easier or more challenging access.

   b. Size
   Various types of phones are available that could "match" the needs of the client (e.g., a cellular phone, larger numbers, dial numbers, or touch tone).

   c. Shape
   The same for size of phone could apply here as well.

   d. Weight
   Again, depending on the type of phone, weight may vary.

   e. Texture
   This is an area that probably does not lend itself to gradation as much as the others.

4. Materials
   a. Position
   n/a

   b. Size
   n/a

c. Shape
n/a

d. Weight
n/a

e. Texture
n/a

5. Nature/Degree of Interpersonal Contact
The nature of the interpersonal contact is indirect in that there is no face-to-face interaction; however, it may still vary in objective or subjective information being exchanged (e.g., a call could be made to a stranger, such as a request for pizza delivery or for a business transaction, or it could be made to a friend or relative with whom the client may feel close).

6. Extent of Tactile, Verbal, or Visual Cues Used by Practitioner During Activity
The practitioner could vary the amount of assistance from maximum cueing and "hands-on" facilitation initially and gradually lessen the physical and cognitive supervision needed for the client to complete the activity independently.

7. The Teaching-Learning Environment
The environment could be adjusted to meet the needs of the client in a variety of ways (e.g., the room itself could be quiet with little distractions or the client could be asked to make the call at a busy traffic intersection on a public pay phone), space and placement of tools could change, from a large desk to a kitchen phone by a small counter.

C. Therapeutic Modifications—Indicate ways in which this activity may be changed to increase occupational performance. State your reasoning. Write "n/a" if not applicable. Definitions for the following terms can be found in Appendix B, *Uniform Terminology for Reporting Occupational Therapy Service, First Edition,* "Therapeutic Adaptations" and "The Guide to O.T. Practice," AOTA, 1999.

1. Therapeutic Adaptations
   a. Orthotic Devices
   If needed, an orthotic device or splint could be created to help the client grasp the receiver.

   b. Prosthetic Devices
   In this case, training with the prosthesis may be necessary for the client to learn to manipulate the pages of a book, receiver, and dialing numbers.

   c. Assistive Technology and Adaptive Devices
      (1) Architectural Modification
      Chair and desk could be ergonomically correct for maintaining posture or work station could be built into an area if space is a consideration.

      (2) Environmental Modification
      The room may need to be carpeted to soften sound or temperature controlled, again, depending on the needs of the client.

      (3) Tool and Equipment Modification (low tech: e.g., reacher; high tech: e.g., computer control devices)
      Enlarged numbers on phone for those who are visually impaired, or a TDD device for those who are hearing impaired, or speaker phone for someone who has difficulty with arm motion and hand/finger manipulation are just some possibilities.

      (4) Wheelchair Modification
      A lap tray can be used instead of a desk, or the wheelchair may require desk arms to fit under the work station. Footrests may need to swing away, or if needed, be adjusted comfortably for feet support.

2. Prevention
  a. Energy Conservation
    (1) Energy-Saving Procedures
    Address book should be at the desk ready for use to avoid having to locate it. The phone number could be in the phone memory so it is accessible by the push of one button instead of 10.

    (2) Activity Restriction
    Client may be asked to restrict himself from making too many calls, which makes him feel fatigued.

    (3) Work Simplification
    As mentioned earlier, using phone memory and having all materials at hand will make the activity simpler for the client.

    (4) Time Management
    In terms of social conduct or endurance, for example, the client may need to be reminded to make calls at only appropriate times or limit calls.

    (5) Environmental Organization
    Items on desk should be organized in such a way that the client can reach them easily. Desk, chair, and phone should be easily accessible for normal use as well as for emergency situations.

  b. Joint Protection/Body Mechanics
    (1) Using Proper Body Mechanics
    Especially for reaching items, client may need to be reminded of proper movement patterns; and for sitting, a chair with good trunk, arm, and leg support is needed. Elbows could rest on desk to keep arms from tiring.

    (2) Avoiding Static/Deforming Postures
    The client may need to be reminded to maintain good body posture and limit use of the phone, providing rest periods as needed.

    (3) Avoiding Excessive Weight-Bearing
    This shouldn't be a problem if the client is sitting while making a call. If standing, proper body mechanics should be emphasized.

  c. Positioning
  Depending upon the placement of the phone, positioning could take on many forms; but no matter if standing or sitting, good body mechanics and ergonomically correct body posture is essential.

  d. Balance of Performance Areas to Facilitate Health and Well-Being
    (1) Enhancement of Occupational Performance Areas
    The areas of functional communication and socialization will be enhanced by the client through this occupational performance.

    (2) Satisfaction of Client and/or Caregiver
    In this case, the client will feel pleased that he has been able to complete a call and converse with a friend.

    (3) Quality of Life
    Feeling good about "doing" an activity by oneself and being in touch with a positive support system contributes to one's well-being.

NOTES

NOTES

NOTES

Unit Seven

CORRELATING THE ACTIVITY

OBJECTIVES

Upon completion of this unit, the student will be able to:

❖ Identify the problem areas from the client's profile to be addressed in occupational therapy.

❖ Prioritize and develop long- and short-term goals that respond to the referral.

❖ Select, describe, prepare, and implement a purposeful activity that addresses improved occupational performance in response to the referral.

❖ Use Uniform Terminology to document the client's performance.

The Client-Activity Correlation demonstrates the relationship between the client's present lack of performance and the meaningful activity selected as the avenue for intervention. While the term "correlation" is often considered a research term, in this setting it is defined as "a mutual relationship or connection" (*Webster's New World College Dictionary*, 1997). A positive correlation occurs if the purposeful activity used in treatment produces responses in the client that are significant in reaching the goals of therapy. A negative correlation occurs if performance of the activity produces a weak or unsatisfactory response. This correlation is illustrated in the Occupational Therapy Process (*American Journal of Occupational Therapy*, 1999), which describes the occupational therapy protocol for treating a client. The Occupational Therapy Process begins with the referral and progresses through the evaluation phase, the development of the intervention plan, the intervention itself and subsequent reevaluation, and concludes with either discharge or further follow-up.

The Client-Activity Correlation addresses the second stage of the Occupational Therapy Process and outlines the development of the intervention plan. It is here that the practitioner and the client together identify realistic and meaningful treatment goals. For the student, the Client-Activity Correlation provides the synthesis of learning that has been building through the use of the Activity Awareness, Action Identification, and Activity Analysis Forms. Now it is time to move into the areas of occupation that are meaningful to the client and appropriate to the development of the client's occupational competence. The Client-Activity Correlation concept provides a five-step organizational framework that demonstrates development of goals, choice of purposeful activity, a preparation sequence, an intervention sequence, and a method of documentation based on Uniform Terminology.

GOALS OF THERAPY

By combining professional expertise and clinical

reasoning with the information gained from the client's referral, evaluation measures, and other professionals, the occupational therapist develops the long- and short-term goals of therapy. These goals denote endpoints of treatment and include the way carefully selected activities will stimulate improvement in the client's occupational performance. The goals and the activities must demonstrate a therapeutic and meaningful correlation with each other and to the client. Each goal and its accompanying purposeful activities must clearly demonstrate the progress the client will be expected to make toward those endpoints.

Long-term goals indicate the expected final outcomes of therapy. The therapist anticipates the client's occupational performance at the projected time of discharge. Long-term goals frequently include a specific period of time or number of treatments. However, current health care guidelines may dictate that therapy will address only some of the client's immediate needs. Intervention may be further constrained by payment for a limited number of treatments. In today's market, the practitioner must continually employ creative and resourceful clinical reasoning skills to effectively address the client's most realistic and immediate goals for increased occupational performance.

Short-term goals are one or more units of accomplishment that must be completed to reach each long-term goal. They are described as a series of blocks of activity that are purposefully selected, sequenced, and graded to lead to the occupational competence defined by the long-term goal. The following example demonstrates how one long-term goal requires the completion of seven short-term goals.

Example

Long-term goal: At discharge, the client will demonstrate independence in routinely using school bus transportation four out of five weekday mornings.

Short-term goals: To demonstrate independence in using school bus transportation, the client will:

1. Self-monitor the time for leaving home.

2. Arrive at the bus stop 5 minutes before the scheduled stop.

3. Dress appropriately for weather conditions.

4. Carry a backpack containing lunch and all required school materials.

5. Board the bus in a sociably accepted manner.

6. Quickly find a vacant seat.

7. Remain seated until the bus driver discharges the students at school.

Both long- and short-term goals have to be observable (student routinely uses the bus successfully), measurable (student arrives at school on time and in a socially acceptable manner at least four out of five days), and expressed in behavioral terms (the client will—). The goals for this client address a major Uniform Terminology performance area (work and productive activities) and are documented using the Uniform Terminology format.

A progress note might read as follows:

Following 2 weeks of occupational therapy intervention, the client successfully demonstrates his independence in using the school bus to get to school on time and in a prepared manner. His parents and teacher have also noted his independence. These goals respond to the Uniform Terminology performance area of activities of daily living (community mobility) and work and production activities (educational activities).

Because accountability, occupational performance, and cost containment are prime criteria for the reimbursement of occupational therapy services, the use of occupation as intervention must be justifiable. When writing either long- or short-term goals, it must be clear that these goals are occupational in intent and are within the guidelines of occupational therapy practice. As in the Activity Analysis Process, Uniform Terminology is used to document the client's level of competence.

The student now begins to realize that each short-term goal is made up of one or more purposeful activities that are used to fulfill the requirements of that goal. Consider the series of activities that are required to complete short-term goal #1.

1. The student will don a watch upon awakening in the morning.

2. The student will frequently check the time while dressing and eating breakfast.

3. The student will understand the time required to cover the distance between home and the bus stop.

4. The student will independently leave home in time to meet the bus.

These four steps define the bus meeting activity required to meet short-term goal #1. The student may realize that each of the four steps listed above could become a goal with its own series of steps embedded in an action sequence.

THE CLIENT-ACTIVITY CORRELATION: AN OVERVIEW

Client Profile and Referral

As in practice, all intervention begins with a referral of a client who will benefit from occupational therapy services. The Client-Activity Correlation Form begins with a brief outline of the client's dysfunction and the referral. The referral information used in preparing the Client-Activity Correlation Form will be more specific than is generally found in practice. This approach is used to narrow the range of goals the student has to consider at this point in the learning process. However, in today's practice, a practitioner frequently finds it necessary to screen the available client population, decide who could benefit from occupational therapy intervention and in what way, and then approach a physician with a request for a referral.

Intervention Goals

Long- and short-term goals are developed from the information found in the client profile and referral. While the need for several long-term goals may be evident, the beginning student should think about the client's most immediate goal. With the meaningful long-term goal firmly in mind, the student can then begin the clinical reasoning process required to analyze the client data and develop the

short-term goals that support that one long-term goal. As the student progresses academically and professionally, the amount of client information readily available through other professional resources will increase.

The student will then be required to discern and prioritize increased opportunities for occupational therapy intervention.

Goal-Directed Purposeful Activity Description

This section requires a brief description of the activity and how it will be used therapeutically. This description is similar to the activity description completed earlier in Section 1 (Activity Summary) of the Activity Analysis Form.

Activity Preparation

Prior to actual contact with the client, the practitioner needs to set aside a block of time to prepare for the therapy session. Consider some or all of the following questions:

❖ What are the goals for this client?

❖ What purposeful activity or activities are appropriate?

❖ What variables need to be considered in arranging the intervention time and place?

❖ How much time will the intervention period require?

❖ What is the client's mental and physical status?

❖ What tools, materials, or equipment are needed in the preparation and where are they located?

❖ Will the preparation take place in the office, the clinic, or another site? How much work space is needed?

❖ How much preparation time is required? Are there specific time lines?

❖ Can the preparation be completed independently? If not, who should assist?

❖ What personal safety precautions should be observed?

For professional credibility, the session should be completed without the distracting frustration that results from insufficient preparation or poor organization on the part of professional personnel. While unforeseen circumstances may sometimes disrupt a treatment session, the habit of thorough preparation is an asset to both the practitioner and the client. Preparation time may be included in the charges for occupational therapy services. Documentation time and consultation with other practitioners or caregivers may also be included.

Activity Implementation

At the appointed time, the client, the therapist, and all required materials and equipment for performing the activity must be in place. Depending on the nature of the activity being used, additional people may need to assist or observe during the treatment session. Co-treating therapists, client caregivers, technicians, vendors, aides, and students are potential personnel. The setting has to be large enough to accommodate all personnel and necessary equipment. Lighting, room temperature, a calming or stimulating atmosphere, privacy issues, and client accessibility to the room or its furnishings are some of the important environmental factors to be considered.

During the session, the therapist also needs to be attuned to the client's physical, cognitive, and psychological condition. If any part of the activity appears to compromise the client's health or safety, the therapist may need to shorten the session or grade and adapt the activity before continuing.

Client-Practitioner Activity Sequence

The expertise of the occupational therapist in using purposeful activity as an agent for change to promote occupational competence is unique to occupational therapy. Clear and concise documentation of the methods and the occupational performance that results are necessary for the client's

records. Therefore, the documentation of the activity sequence used must be more than a listing of a series of steps resembling ingredients in a cookbook. In the Action Identification Form, the student used the Do-What-How format to document the action observed in oneself or by another. In the Client-Activity Correlation, the student expands the Do-What-How concept by adding two more elements from Uniform Terminology: "with what" (performance components) and "under what circumstances" (performance contexts). The student is already familiar with both the performance components and the performance contexts as they were used in the Activity Analysis Form. Return to the example of activities used by the young client learning to use school bus transportation and identify statements that indicate this Do-What-How, With What and Under What Circumstances approach. Is the short-term goal #1 fulfilled?

The therapist documents the major steps of the activity and indicates its therapeutic value. The major steps performed by the client reveal the therapeutic value, not the incidental ones. If the activity contains more than a few steps that are not of therapeutic value or the practitioner must do most of an activity for the client, then a more relevant activity should be chosen. Generally, the therapeutic steps of an activity can be documented in 10 steps or less. It is important to clearly identify the role of the practitioner throughout the intervention. The documentation should demonstrate how the presence and expertise of an occupational therapy practitioner is required to successfully complete the intervention and should be stated in behavioral terms. In thinking about the example of the telephone call that has been used in the previous four forms, a note stated in behavioral terms and demonstrating the role of the practitioner would read:

Given verbal instruction and hand-over-hand guidance by the practitioner, the client will accurately dial a phone number with his non-dominant hand.

Uniform Terminology Documentation

The final section of the Client-Activity Correlation is the use of Uniform Terminology to document the therapy outcomes. This documentation should reflect how the activity generated a change in the client's occupational performance as required in the referral. Proof of this change demonstrates effective occupational intervention and is documented through the use of the performance areas, performance components, and performance contexts of Uniform Terminology. Consider again the young client working on using school bus transportation.

I. *Performance Areas*
   A. *Activities of Daily Living*
      13. *Community Mobility*
   B. *Work and Productive Activities*
      3. *Educational Activities*

II. *Performance Components*
   B. *Cognitive Integration and Cognitive Components*
      4. *Attention Span*
      5. *Initiation of the Activity*
      8. *Sequencing*
      12. *Problem Solving*
   C. *Psychosocial Skills and Psychological Components*
      2. *Social*
         a. *Role Performance*
         b. *Social Conduct*
      3. *Self-Management*
         c. *Self-Control*

III. *Performance Contexts*
   A. *Temporal Aspects*
      1. *Chronological*
      2. *Developmental*
      3. *Life Cycle*

The student is cautioned to use only the portions of Uniform Terminology that actually identify the client's responses to the stated goals. Frequently, students using the Client-Activity Correlation for the first time revert back to the Activity Analysis format that requires a response to all items required to perform an activity. Justification for the use of each item is not required with this form.

DISCUSSION QUESTIONS

1. Why is it important to consider an observable connection (correlation) between what you plan as therapeutic intervention and the problems the client is presenting.

2. Name three of your own long-term goals. How do you plan to achieve them?

3. Based on the information in this chapter, think of ways you might increase your own organizational skill to smooth your daily schedule.

REFERENCES

American Occupational Therapy Association (1994). Uniform terminology for occupational therapy (3rd ed.). *American Journal of Occupational Therapy*, 48(11).

Moyers, P. (1999). The guide to occupational therapy practice. [Special issue]. *American Journal of Occupational Therapy*, 53(3).

Webster's New World College Dictionary (3rd ed.). (1997). USA: Macmillan.

Form 5

CLIENT-ACTIVITY CORRELATION FORM

Student: Example_____ Date: _____

Activity: Making a telephone call_____

Course: _____

1. Client Profile and Referral

Client Information: *The client is a 67-year-old male who is progressively losing his sight due to complications of diabetes. He is now 2 years post-retirement from his position as a senior clergyman in a large local church. Upon retirement, and because of his diminishing vision, he requested permission to initiate a phone ministry to the homebound members of his church. His duties include weekly phone calls to approximately 40 elderly or disabled members to provide social contact, church information, or arrange assistance when necessary. He worked from a small office in his church. He was successful in keeping in touch with members who came to depend on his weekly call. When his failing vision reduced his community mobility, the church members looked for a way for him to continue his ministry from his home.*

At the time of the referral, the client could no longer drive his car or safely walk the three blocks from his home to his office at the church. Public transportation was inadequate. He has a large, sunny study in the first floor of his home, which he now shares with a large parrot and an old Siamese cat. His wife is deceased 3 years. He has been referred to occupational therapy for evaluation and assistance in converting part of his study into a home office. He needs to use the phone independently and be able to record information because he no longer has the assistance of the church secretary.

Referral: *Evaluate and treat for developing independence in using the telephone and for recording incoming information in ways that are compatible with his diminishing vision.*

2. Intervention Goals

a. Long-Term Goal

Together with the practitioner, the client will develop an office arrangement in his home study that will permit him to continue his role as phone minister to the elderly and disabled members of his church. This will include the development of an accessible and functional work station, a safe room arrangement, and the selection and placement of assistive technology to support his independence in phone communication skills, which are now threatened by his progressive loss of vision.

b. Short-Term Goal

The client will independently call one of his parishioners from his new office telephone.

3. Goal-Directed Purposeful Activity Description

The client will experiment with several types of telephones equipped with assistive technological features to find one that best fits his needs. The practitioner will provide the phone samples for testing.

4. Activity Preparation

a. Review Goals, Describe Practitioner's Role

In view of the goals stated above, the practitioner will survey professional technology catalogs to determine the types of phones currently on the market. The practitioner will also confer with the assistive technology staff of the large state rehabilitation center in a neighboring city for further information. With the permission of the technology staff, the practitioner will arrange to borrow three different styles of telephones for 1 week to determine the client's independent use before a permanent purchase is made. The practitioner will carefully learn to use all of the features of each phone before meeting with the client as well as seek resources for funding the purchase of the telephone.

The practitioner will arrange an appointment with the client at his home 3 weeks from today.

b. Personnel Required to Do the Preparation

One practitioner.

c. Required Preparation Time

Approximately 2 weeks.

d. Required Place and Space
The practitioner will work from the clinic office.

e. Materials
Office supplies.

f. Equipment
Desk, chair, telephone, phone book, catalogs.

g. Safety Precautions for Personnel
None required.

5. Activity Implementation
a. Personnel
Client and practitioner.

b. Setting and Location
Client's home study.

c. Space Required
Easy access to and around the client's work station (desk).

d. Environment
Quiet and undisturbed: remove parrot (noise factor) and cat (curiosity). Lighting of the work station and room temperature should be at comfortable levels.

e. Materials
None required.

f. Equipment: Assistive Devices or Adaptations Included
Equipment will include clear desktop space, two chairs, three assistive telephones, convenient wall jack for phone, and a rolling card file with names and phone numbers in large print.

g. Required Intervention Time
One and one-half hours. In addition to setting up the equipment and trying each phone, the client and practitioner need time to thoroughly consider the features of each and have ample opportunity to try them as often as necessary.

h. Safety Precautions for Client
There should be an unobstructed pathway from the doorway of the study to the chair at the desk. The desk should be free of clutter. The three phones should be within easy reach to facilitate easy comparison.

6. Client-Practitioner Activity Sequence (10 action steps or less)
  1. *The client will seat himself at his desk.*
  2. *The practitioner will place one phone on the desk within the comfortable working range of the client.*
  3. *After determining the phone to be in working order, the practitioner will verbally and tactilely describe the working features.*
  4. *The client will then follow the practitioner's directions in using each feature.*
  5. *The practitioner will observe the ergonomic aspects of the client's use of the phone and make recommendations for increasing his work comfort and efficiency.*
  6. *This sequence will be repeated for the other two phones.*
  7. *The client and practitioner will then spend sufficient time evaluating the positive and negative features of each phone to determine the one that offers him the most independence.*
  8. *After the client makes his selection, he will select a name and number from his card file and successfully call a waiting client.*

7. Uniform Terminology Documentation

 I. *Performance Areas*

  A. *Activities of Daily Living*

   11. *Functional Communication*

  B. *Work and Productive Activities*

   4. *Vocational Activities*

    c. *Work or Job Performance*

 II. *Performance Components*

  A. *Sensorimotor Components*

   1. *Sensory*

    a. *Sensory Awareness*

     (1) *Tactile*

  C. *Psychosocial Skills and Psychological Components*

   2. *Social*

    a. *Role Performance*

 III. *Performance Contexts*

  A. *Temporal Aspects*

   4. *Disability Status*

  B. *Environmental Aspects*

   1. *Physical*

NOTES

NOTES

NOTES

Module IV

THE VERSATILITY OF ACTIVITY

Throughout the first three modules, the use of activity as an instrument for change has been demonstrated in numerous ways. Activity performance has surfaced from the unconscious and demanded attention. The required steps of an activity have been graded, adapted, added to, reduced, and rearranged. Activity is viewed as a universal requirement for meaningful life.

In the second and third modules, the simple activity of making a phone call was utilized as a teaching tool to develop the progressive understanding and use of the five forms presented in the text. The phone call activity was first called to consciousness, reduced to its components and context, then reassembled with its therapeutic implications. Finally, it was used as treatment in an occupational setting for an adult individual.

In Module IV, Unit Eight, a simple activity has again been used sequentially in all five of the forms. These examples are used to further illustrate the versatility of activity as occupational therapy intervention. In the first four forms, the activity is examined as before. This time the fifth form, the application portion of the process, demonstrates the use of a goal-directed activity in a group therapy situation. In this example, the elements of a cookie baking activity are organized by the practitioner to facilitate an increase in the socialization skills of a small group of young school children.

Finally, Unit Nine provides information for the student to download all five of the forms used in this text from a companion website. Since the forms will be able to be saved onto a computer hard drive or disk, this will allow the student to have easy access to all or part of each of the forms as class assignments require; the forms can be used easily and often. This makes activity analysis and its application to intervention a portable educational tool that can be used in the classroom, in fieldwork, and eventually in the workplace. The student will find value in its use for documentation, education of clients and staff, and ergonomic evaluations, just to name a few opportunities for use. Use of the downloaded forms as an effective reporting and demonstration tool can further demonstrate the range of occupational therapy services to the public.

Unit Eight

REVIEWING THE PROCESS

Form I

ACTIVITY AWARENESS FORM

Student: <u>Example</u>   Date: _____

Activity: <u>Making cookies from a recipe</u>

Course: _____

Directions: Reflecting on the activity just performed, complete the following sentences with the first words that come to mind.

1. During this activity I was thinking about... *the times my Mom and I would make cookies as a kid.*

2. While doing this activity I felt... *I should do this more often. It's a lot of fun.*

3. In doing this activity, the parts of my body I remember using were... *my fingers and hands, my tongue to taste, my nose to smell.*

4. To do this activity I need to... *pay attention so I don't add the wrong ingredient or leave the pans in the oven too long.*

5. When I do this activity again I will... *set it up at a counter with chairs so we can all sit down to work. Also I would make a double recipe.*

6. From doing this activity I became aware of... *how much I enjoy baking, especially the smells and eating homemade items.*

Form 2

ACTION IDENTIFICATION FORM

Student: <u>Example</u>   Date: _____

Activity: <u>Making cookies from a recipe</u>

Course: _____

Directions: Select an activity, and using the Do-What-How style, list the major actions in sequence in 10 steps or less required for you to perform this activity. Repeat the exercise after observing someone else performing the same activity.

OBSERVATION OF SELF

1. Assemble the recipe ingredients appropriately.
2. Measure out the ingredients and mix them up thoroughly.
3. Preheat the oven correctly.
4. Grease the cookie sheets sparingly.
5. Spoon and drop the dough on the sheet spacing leniently.
6. Put filled sheets in the oven and set the timer accurately.
7. Wait for the cookies to bake patiently.
8. Remove sheets and put cookies on wax paper carefully.
9. Wash up dishes and counter completely.
10. Eat cookies eagerly.

OBSERVATION OF ANOTHER

1. Read the directions thoughtfully.
2. Find and lay out the ingredients and utensils thoroughly.
3. Preheat the oven and prepare the trays accurately.
4. Follow the recipe carefully.
5. Place the dough on the trays appropriately.
6. Put the trays in to bake and set the time correctly.
7. Set the dishes to soak efficiently.
8. Remove the cookies cautiously.
9. Clean the dishes and kitchen area completely.
10. Sit down and eat cookies contentedly.

Form 3

ACTIVITY ANALYSIS FOR EXPECTED PERFORMANCE

Student: <u>Example</u>   Date: _____

Activity: <u>Making cookies from a recipe</u>

Course: _____

SECTION I: ACTIVITY SUMMARY

Directions: Respond to the following in list format.

1. Name of Activity

Making cookies from a recipe.

2. Brief Description of Activity

The student will read the recipe directions for chocolate chip cookies, gather necessary tools and ingredients, prepare dough according to recipe directions, and bake cookies.

3. Tools/Equipment (non-expendable), Cost, and Source

The tools and equipment needed for baking cookies can be purchased in the housewares department of a retail establishment. These items include:

Mixing bowl, $3.00

Mixing spoon, $1.00

Measuring cups, $1.00

Baking sheet, $3.00

Cooling racks, $3.00

Spatula, $1.00

Oven mitt, $3.00

An oven with a built-in timer (on hand, no recent cost expended). The total cost for non-expendable tools and equipment is $15.00.

4. Materials/Supplies (expendable), Cost, and Source

The ingredients necessary for making chocolate chip cookies can be purchased at a grocery store. Materials and supplies needed include:

Flour

Eggs

Granulated white sugar

Brown sugar

Salt

Butter

Chocolate chip morsels

Also, gas or electric energy is required to operate the oven. The total cost for expendable items is less than $10.00.

5. Space/Environmental Requirements

To perform this activity, it is necessary to have a kitchen facility with adequate counter space (approximately 5 feet).

6. Sequence of Major Steps (in 10 steps or less; specify time required to complete each step)

    1. *Read recipe directions, 2 min.*

    2. *Gather necessary ingredients and utensils (assuming they are already available in kitchen), 5 min.*

    3. *Preset oven temperature, 30 sec.*

    4. *Measure and mix ingredients, 10 min.*

    5. *Place mixed dough on baking sheet, 5 min.*

6. *Place baking sheet in the oven, 1 min.*
7. *Set oven timer, 30 sec.*
8. *Allow cookies to bake in oven, 15 min.*
9. *Remove baking sheet from oven, 1 min.*
10. *Remove cookies from baking sheet and place on cooling racks, 5 min.*
Total amount of time needed to bake cookies is approximately 45 minutes.

7. Precautions (review "Sequence of Major Steps")
When baking cookies, the student should use an oven mitt upon placing the baking sheet in or when removing the sheet from the oven. It is important that an oven mitt also be used while removing the cookies from a hot baking sheet. Also, it is important that the student understands the proper safety procedures used when operating an oven and that quantities of ingredients or baking temperatures should not be altered.

8. Special Considerations (age appropriateness, educational requirements, cultural relevance, gender identification, other)
To complete this activity, the student must be able to read, comprehend mathematical concepts such as fractions, and be capable of operating an oven. No set gender identification needs to be made. Culturally, the person would value and have an interest in cooking and preparing food for self or others. In many subgroups of society, this activity is highly looked upon and respected.

9. Acceptable Criteria for Completed Project
The finished product of this activity are cookies that are golden brown, edible and tasty, and of an appropriate size to be eaten by hand.

SECTION 2: ANALYZING OCCUPATIONAL PERFORMANCE AREAS, COMPONENTS, AND CONTEXTS

Part I. Performance Areas
A. Activities of Daily Living
1. Grooming
n/a

2. Oral Hygiene
n/a

3. Bathing/Showering
n/a

4. Toilet Hygiene
n/a

5. Personal Device Care
n/a

6. Dressing
n/a

7. Feeding and Eating
Cookies will be eaten following preparation and baking.

8. Medication Routine
n/a

9. Health Maintenance
Cooking and baking could be considered a survival skill; however, in this case, they are being prepared for mostly leisure and social reasons.

10. Socialization
Giving cookies to another may be considered a way of interacting and sharing with another. Also, cookies could be prepared in a group setting.

11. Functional Communication
n/a

12. Functional Mobility
Moving about the kitchen to retrieve tools and ingredients for cooking and baking purposes is considered a type of functional mobility.

13. Community Mobility
n/a

14. Emergency Response
n/a

15. Sexual Expression
n/a

B. Work and Productive Activities
1. Home Management
   a. Clothing Care
n/a

   b. Cleaning
n/a

   c. Meal Preparation/Cleanup
The student will prepare cookies, open and close containers, use an oven, and manipulate kitchen utensils. Cleanup will take place as well.

   d. Shopping
The student may need to shop for ingredients, but for this particular activity, all ingredients were available in the kitchen.

   e. Money Management
It is possible that when purchasing ingredients, the student will need to be aware of the cost of items. If there is a limited budget, generic or store brands could serve as an alternative to more expensive name brands.

   f. Household Maintenance
To perform a baking activity, the student will want to ensure that all equipment (e.g., oven, refrigerator, water faucets, etc.) are in a safe and working order.

   g. Safety Procedures
Safety is part of this activity when using kitchen utensils and oven.

2. Care of Others
n/a

3. Educational Activities
n/a

4. Vocational Activities
   a. Vocational Exploration
   n/a

   b. Job Acquisition
   n/a

   c. Work or Job Performance
   n/a

   d. Retirement Planning
   n/a

   e. Volunteer Participation
   n/a

C. Play or Leisure Activities
1. Play or Leisure Exploration
n/a

2. Play or Leisure Performance
Baking cookies may serve as a leisure skill for the student, providing an enjoyable activity to the person.

Part II. Performance Components

A. Sensorimotor Components
1. Sensory
   a. Sensory Awareness
   I am aware of many incoming sensory stimuli, such as olfactory, visual, auditory, gustatory, movement, and environmental variables, as I perform this activity.

   b. Sensory Processing
      (1) Tactile
      This sense comes about through touch made with the tools and ingredients.

      (2) Proprioceptive
      I can sense the position of my body motions in relation to the counter top, tools, oven, and ingredients (e.g., in stirring the batter, my hand to the spoon and to the bowl on the counter space).

      (3) Vestibular
      I am able to stand upright, move about the work area, and change positions while performing this activity.

      (4) Visual
      I see all about me and can identify the ingredients; read the recipe, time, and temperature dials; and judge the doneness of the cookies by sight.

      (5) Auditory
      I hear the ring of the oven timer and know that is the signal that the cookies are done and should be taken out of oven.

(6) Gustatory

I may sneak a taste of the batter and, of course, taste the cookies when they are done.

(7) Olfactory

The ingredients can be smelled to discern their freshness, and the cookies can be smelled while they are baking.

c. Perceptual Processing

(1) Stereognosis

I am able to reach for an object that I want on the counter space while paying attention to what I'm mixing in the bowl.

(2) Kinesthesia

I'm aware of the movement of my arms and legs as I mix the dough, stand at the counter, place pans in the oven, and remove pans from the oven.

(3) Pain Response

If I burn myself on the oven or pans, the pain response is immediate.

(4) Body Scheme

As I move about the kitchen and perform this activity, I'm aware of my body parts moving in relation to others (e.g., arm mixing the bowl close to my trunk or bending at the waist to place pans in oven).

(5) Right-Left Discrimination

As I mix the ingredients, I use both sides of my body (e.g., holding the vanilla bottle in the left and measuring spoon in the right, or knowing the oven is on the left side of the counter and the pantry is on the right).

(6) Form Constancy

I recognize that the form of the unbaked cookie is about the same as after it is baked (i.e., round and flat). The measuring cups and bowls will be the same no matter if sitting on the shelf or filled with ingredients.

(7) Position in Space

I sense my position and its distance from the counter top and oven so that I can work efficiently.

(8) Visual-Closure

Even though the dough is of a different consistency and incomplete, I recognize that it will be a cookie once baked. I can envision its size, taste, and smell!

(9) Figure Ground

The baker is able to distinguish the ingredients and utensils from the counter space, and when I read the recipe, I see letters on the page accurately.

(10) Depth Perception

I am aware of the distance objects are from me, how far back in the oven the cookie pans are placed, and how deep the mixing bowls are.

(11) Spatial Relations

Again, I am aware of objects and their distance from me and each other (e.g., the ingredients sit alongside the bowl and spatula, the oven mitt is next to the oven for easy reach).

(12) Topographical Orientation

Being able to find my way around the kitchen and to locate utensils is an example of this kind of perception.

2. Neuromusculoskeletal
  a. Reflex
  Because my reflexes are integrated, I am able to move about voluntarily; but if a pain response is necessary, my withdrawal response will come into immediate action.

  b. Range of Motion
  Active range of motion is needed to move the upper and lower extremities while performing this activity (e.g., shoulder flexion and extension for reaching, hand flexion and extension for grasping objects).

  c. Muscle Tone
  Sufficient muscle tone is needed to control the movements of mixing and holding ingredients as well as standing while at work.

  d. Strength
  Fair plus to normal strength is needed to lift ingredients, mix the dough, and maintain an erect posture.

  e. Endurance
  I need enough stamina to begin and complete the activity in the time allotted.

  f. Postural Control
  It is necessary for me to maintain a standing posture while mixing the cookie dough at the counter and use proper posture while placing items in and removing items from the oven.

  g. Postural Alignment
  In order to maintain good body mechanics, such as when bending at knees instead of waist when placing cookies in oven, I need to keep my trunk in good alignment with other parts of my body.

  h. Soft Tissue Integrity
  To protect tissue, I must be cautious around the hot oven to avoid burning myself.

3. Motor
  a. Gross Coordination
  Large muscle groups at shoulder, trunk, and hips are under active control in order for me to move around the kitchen, mix the dough, carry the pans, and stand upright.

  b. Crossing the Midline
  The midline is crossed when reaching to locate items across the counter space and when mixing the dough.

  c. Laterality
  I use my right dominant hand to handle most activities.

  d. Bilateral Integration
  Both upper extremities are used to mix the dough and to place cookie pans in and remove them from the oven.

  e. Motor Control
  While cooking, I need sufficient motor control to move my body through the various movement patterns of the activity.

  f. Praxis
  Baking cookies could be a new motor act for me, in which case I need to conceive and plan how to perform the activity. Or, even if I know how to bake, I may be challenged by a new demand in the environment and respond with a new or unrehearsed motor act (e.g., sufficient chocolate chips are unavailable as I had thought, so I add crushed nuts that are on hand to fill in the batter).

g. Fine Coordination/Dexterity
Throughout this activity, fine coordination of hand and fingers are in high demand as I measure ingredients, manipulate utensils, and place cookie dough on the pans.

h. Visual-Motor Integration
Again, throughout this activity, my hands and eyes are constantly working together in order to complete the activity.

i. Oral-Motor Control
Ah, yes, what a wonderful taste!

B. Cognitive Integration and Cognitive Components

1. Level of Arousal
This is essential when working in the kitchen and handling ingredients for predetermined quantities and being cognizant of safety concerns.

2. Orientation
I know who I am, the time of day, and where I am in order to complete this activity (e.g., I'm an adult who is making cookies for a friend; it's morning and I have sufficient time to complete the activity before going to class; and I'm in the appropriate room of the house—the kitchen—in order to complete the activity effectively).

3. Recognition
I am familiar with all tools and ingredients needed for activity completion.

4. Attention Span
I am able to focus on the activity for the allotted time necessary.

5. Initiation of Activity
It is apparent to me when I can start this activity, as I know the time, feel motivated, and have the needed ingredients to begin.

6. Termination of Activity
I know that there is only a certain amount of time to complete the activity and am aware that when the cookies are done baking and I've cleaned up after myself, the activity can be considered finished.

7. Memory
Short-term memory is used to recall the recipe and the ingredients, the sequence of the activity directions, the time required to bake the cookies, and when to check on cookies baking in the oven.

8. Sequencing
I need to be able to place information and actions in order to complete the activity so that cookies are properly prepared (e.g., I need to grease the cookie pans before placing the cookies by spoonful onto the cookie pan for baking).

9. Categorization
It is necessary to understand the difference between wet and dry ingredients and of substitutions that can be made, for instance, margarine for butter or caramel chips for chocolate chips.

10. Concept Formation
I have an idea of what cookies taste and look like based on prior experience of baking and eating them.

11. Spatial Operations
I am able to manipulate the bowl and the cookie pans according to their use during the process of baking.

12. Problem Solving
This process occurs throughout the preparation and baking process. For example, I taste and look at the dough to determine if the ingredients are fresh and in proper proportion to one another. I may also need to determine when substitutions of ingredients are needed or how to correct errors with baking times and varying oven temperatures.

13. Learning
Acquiring new ideas about baking may take place (e.g., the cookies are burned and I realize the oven temperature is inaccurate and needs adjustment so that next time that is prevented from happening, or I realize that I can make substitutions in the recipe and the cookies taste even better).

14. Generalization
Mathematical and reading skills and previous knowledge of oven and utensil use are helpful when confronted with this baking activity.

C. Psychosocial Skills and Psychological Components
1. Psychological
a. Values
I value my friendship and wish to share cookies with my friend as a token and gift of our friendship.

b. Interests
Baking is an interest of mine which I enjoy doing.

c. Self-Concept
Baking cookies gives me a sense of satisfaction knowing that I can perform this activity well.

2. Social
a. Role Performance
Baking cookies for others is compatible with the student's role of friend.

b. Social Conduct
I am working alone in the kitchen so interacting with others is not a consideration.

c. Interpersonal Skills
Again, I am not interacting with others, but the cookies will serve as a nonverbal, nonhuman way of expressing my friendship.

d. Self-Expression
By making the cookies, I'm expressing my skill in baking as well as in creativity by varying the recipe.

3. Self-Management
a. Coping Skills
I may need to cope when an unexpected event occurs (e.g., making an error in the order of the ingredients).

b. Time Management
The student must allocate sufficient amount of time to prepare and bake cookies.

c. Self-Control
The student must appropriately react to problem situations as they arise, such as running out of ingredients or over-baking the cookies.

Part III. Performance Contexts

A. Temporal Aspects
1. Chronological
I am 24 years of age.

2. Developmental
Making cookies from a recipe is an age-appropriate activity, as it is an activity that can be work- or leisure-related.

3. Life Cycle
Because I am in the stage of young adulthood, the activity is appropriate as it requires reading competence, following directions, and having knowledge of basic kitchen safety skills.

4. Disability Status
n/a

B. Environmental Aspects
1. Physical
The activity takes place in a kitchen so that I have access to the oven, sink, counter space, refrigerator, proper utensils, and ingredients.

2. Social
I am working alone.

3. Cultural
Baking cookies is a valued activity of my cultural group of peers and family, and one that is looked upon positively.

Form 4

ACTIVITY ANALYSIS FOR THERAPEUTIC INTERVENTION

Student: <u>Example</u>   Date: _____

Activity: <u>Making cookies from a recipe</u>

Course: _____

SECTION 1: ACTIVITY DESCRIPTION

A. Provide a Brief Description of Activity

The student will read the recipe directions for chocolate chip cookies, gather necessary tools and ingredients, prepare dough according to recipe directions, and bake cookies.

B. Identify Major Steps
 1. *Read recipe directions.*
 2. *Gather necessary ingredients and utensils.*
 3. *Preset oven temperature.*
 4. *Measure and mix ingredients.*
 5. *Place mixed dough on baking sheet.*
 6. *Place baking sheet in the oven.*
 7. *Set oven timer.*
 8. *Allow cookies to bake in oven.*
 9. *Remove baking sheet from oven.*
 10. *Remove cookies from baking sheet and place on cooling rack.*

SECTION 2: THERAPEUTIC QUALITIES

A. Energy Patterns—Describe the required energy level in terms of light, moderate, or heavy work patterns and provide an explanation for the level specified.

A moderate work pattern is used to complete this activity. The person needs to be sufficiently focused and organized to prepare and complete the activity as well as physically able to move about in the setting and to handle the utensils and equipment. Both cognitive and physical demands are placed upon the person but they are not physically or mentally exhausting.

B. Activity Patterns—Indicate the patterns of the activity expected for successful completion of the activity.

1. Structural/Methodical/Orderly

Making cookies has all three characteristics, as the person must follow the steps listed in the recipe, be able to break an egg, know how to measure, and maintain some order to the process so ingredients are not used in error and the kitchen is kept somewhat clean and neat.

2. Repetitive

The steps of mixing the dough, dropping dough by spoonfuls onto cookie pan, and removing cookies one by one from the pan all have a repetitive pattern to them.

3. Expressive/Creative/Projective

The person expresses his friendship and giving through the art of making cookies; one could easily be creative with substitution in the dough mix and with decorating cookies.

4. Tactile
   a. Contact with Others (e.g., hands-on, stand by assist)
   As the activity is being performed, there is no contact with others.

b. Materials (e.g., pliable, sensual)
While performing this activity, there is the feel of the dough which is soft and pliable to the touch, or of other ingredients which may be liquid or solid.

c. Equipment (e.g., size, manageability, shape)
In doing this activity, the person handles the utensils, oven, refrigerator, and counter top. Typically, these tools and equipment are of the correct size and shape for managing most kitchen tasks.

SECTION 3: THERAPEUTIC APPLICATION

A. Population—Discuss for whom and in what way increased occupational performance can be derived from the use of this activity. Consider the sensorimotor, cognitive, and psychosocial aspects. Identify any contraindications.
This activity falls in Performance Areas of Activities of Daily Living: Socialization and Functional Mobility; Work and Productive Activities: Home Management, Meal Preparation/Cleanup, and Safety Procedures. Depending upon its purpose, it could be considered Play or Leisure Performance if being done as a leisure activity by the person.
This kind of activity lends itself to almost all the Performance Components; however, it specifically is useful with the following sensorimotor components: Tactile, Gustatory, Olfactory, Kinesthesia, Position in Space, Endurance, Postural Control, Crossing the Midline, Praxis, and Fine Motor Coordination/Dexterity; cognition components: Memory, Sequencing, Problem Solving, and Generalization; and psychosocial components: Values, Interests, Role Performance, and Time Management.
Contraindications may be indicated for those who cognitively cannot grasp safety procedures or for those who may be self-destructive with utensils/tools. Also, any clients with a contagious illness may need to be excluded. Being aware of food allergies and clients with diabetes or any food-restricted diet will need to be considered. It is possible that substitutions could be made.
Population-based groups for which this activity may have applicability are: stroke and geriatric clients for training in an activity of daily living and homemaking or a confidence builder for clients with psychosocial deficits.
Anyone requiring standing tolerance and endurance would be appropriate.
This activity can also be used for persons with brain injuries who need to practice activity planning and following directions. This activity has applicability to almost every age group, from preschool through adulthood, as it can be adapted in a variety of ways to "fit" the needs of the client group. Its versatility is what makes it so appealing for many types of clinical and community settings.

B. Gradation—Describe ways to grade this activity in terms of:

1. Activity Sequence, Duration, and/or the Activity Procedures
The sequence of the activity can be altered to match the needs of the client in a variety of ways (e.g., using a boxed cookie mix or even refrigerator cookie mix to lessen the steps; the amount of supervision can vary from hands-on to observation only). Duration of activity can be shortened or broken into short periods of rest, if needed by the client, depending on the person's endurance, attention span, or capabilities.
Activity procedure can be graded, as above, with different kinds of recipes presented to client; other possibilities are using an electric mixer instead of a spoon to mix, having all ingredients pre-measured, or having the practitioner place the cookie pans in the oven instead of client for safety concerns. To eliminate the hazard of oven use, there are non-baking cookie recipes.

2. Working Position of the Individual
The client can sit, stand, or alternate the two at the work station to prepare the dough.

3. Tools
   a. Position
   The cooking utensils could be placed at different sites on the counter for easier or more challenging reach. However, the layout of the kitchen equipment will dictate accessibility.

   b. Size
   Bowl size could vary for easier handling.

c. Shape
Shape of handles of utensils may be varied for easier grasp.

d. Weight
Mixing bowls and spatula could be weighted for easier handling.

e. Texture
This is an area that probably does not lend itself to gradation as much as the others.

4. Materials
  a. Position
Ingredients could be pre-measured for easier access or the client may be asked to retrieve ingredients independently.

  b. Size
Larger or smaller amounts of cookie dough could be made depending again on the purpose of the activity.

  c. Shape
Drop cookies could vary in shape; cookie dough could be rolled out and cut with cookie cutters.

  d. Weight
Uniform and about 1 tablespoon full.

  e. Texture
The nature of the dough could be altered to be more crunchy or smooth, depending on the recipe and desired taste.

5. Nature/Degree of Interpersonal Contact
Interpersonal contact could be graded from a solitary act to a group activity. Supervision could vary from hands-on, guided, or stand-by depending on needs of the client.

6. Extent of Tactile, Verbal, or Visual Cues Used by Practitioner During Activity
The practitioner could vary the amount of assistance from maximum cueing and "hands-on" facilitation initially and gradually lessen the physical and cognitive supervision needed for the client to complete the activity independently. Directions could be given verbally, by demonstration, or by pictures or a combination of these methods.

7. The Teaching-Learning Environment
The environment of the kitchen setting could vary from a simulated kitchen in a clinic; a mock-up work area with table, chair, and utensils only; or an actual home visit. The area could be graded from distraction-free to the typical noise of a clinic. Again, depending upon the needs of the client, the teaching-learning possibilities vary.

C. Therapeutic Modifications—Indicate ways in which this activity may be changed to increase occupational performance. State your reasoning. Write "n/a" if not applicable. Definitions for the following terms can be found in Appendix B, *Uniform Terminology for Reporting Occupational Therapy Services, First Edition,* "Therapeutic Adaptations" and "The Guide to O.T. Practice," AOTA, 1999.

1. Therapeutic Adaptations
  a. Orthotic Devices
If needed, an orthotic device or splint could be created to help the client grasp the spatula or spoon.

  b. Prosthetic Devices
Meal preparation provides the client with either an upper or lower extremity prosthesis to practice skills (e.g., for the upper extremity amputation, making cookies demands the person use the prosthesis with a variety of utensils, and for the lower extremity amputation, standing tolerance is facilitated).

c. Assistive Technology and Adaptive Devices
(1) Architectural Modification
This is an area in which more or less modification could be done in the kitchen to facilitate or challenge the person, again depending upon the purpose of the activity and the needs of the client. For example, a work station at wheelchair height could be built instead of using a counter top. Or, cabinets could have pull-out drawers and turn tables for easier access.

(2) Environmental Modification
Flooring, space, lighting, and temperature are all considerations.

(3) Tool and Equipment Modification (low tech: e.g., reacher; high tech: e.g., computer control devices)
Several kinds of adaptations can be made to the tools and equipment (e.g., mixer stand, built-up handles, a cart to carry cookie pans to oven, a ledge on the counter top to prevent items from moving during preparation, a suction cup, Dycem, or a coiled damp towel to hold the measuring cup or the mixing bowl).

(4) Wheelchair Modification
A wheelchair tray could be attached for easier handling of the utensils if a counter top is inaccessible. Leg rests that swing away and desk arms allow the person closer access to the work station.

2. Prevention
   a. Energy Conservation
(1) Energy-Saving Procedures
Having all utensils and ingredients at hand lessens exertion.
Sitting while mixing the dough, breaking the activity down into smaller steps, preparing the dough first and refrigerating it, then later completing baking, are energy-saving options.

(2) Activity Restriction
As noted above, the activity can be broken down into smaller steps, rest breaks can be provided, and the activity can be divided into preparation and baking stages.

(3) Work Simplification
An electric mixer could be used to simplify the activity of mixing, or again the activity could be broken down into smaller steps. Assistance could be provided as needed.

(4) Time Management
To conserve time, the ingredients and supplies could be gathered at one time. Making cookies should be done at a time that allows for all steps to be completed, or plan ahead how best to divide the activity into stages so one could be delayed without spoiling prepared dough.

(5) Environmental Organization
Supplies and ingredients could be gathered and placed together on the counter space before preparation is started. Working in a kitchen area that allows for easy access to supplies and ingredients needs to be considered.

b. Joint Protection/Body Mechanics
(1) Using Proper Body Mechanics
During the performance of the activity, the client should use proper body mechanics such as bending from the knees instead of the waist, not overstretching to reach for items from cabinets, and if sitting at the work station, have a chair with good trunk, leg, and foot support.

(2) Avoiding Static/Deforming Postures
Work surface height should be appropriate for standing or sitting while making cookies.

(3) Avoiding Excessive Weight-Bearing
This should be monitored by the practitioner, especially if the client has limited standing tolerance or low endurance.

c. Positioning
The activity can be done in a sitting or standing position; either way, the practitioner should make sure that the client has sufficient support and body mechanics.

d. Balance of Performance Areas to Facilitate Health and Well-Being
   (1) Enhancement of Occupational Performance Areas
   The areas of meal preparation, functional mobility, and possibly leisure performance will be enhanced by performing this activity.

   (2) Satisfaction of Client and/or Caregiver
   The client will be happy with the completion of this activity and being able to share the cookies with a friend. Positive self-concept is a likely outcome.

   (3) Quality of Life
   Receiving satisfaction from completing such an activity as making cookies contributes to one's well-being, as it provides a sense of accomplishment and social connection in gift giving.

Form 5

CLIENT-ACTIVITY CORRELATION FORM

Student: <u>Example</u>   Date: _____

Activity: <u>Making cookies from a recipe</u>

Course: _____

1. Client Profile and Referral

The occupational therapist assigned to School #27 is working weekly with a group of five third-graders who have multiple disabilities. Two have learning disabilities, one has Down syndrome, one has attention deficit disorder, and the fifth has osteogenesis imperfecta and uses a wheelchair. These children have been working on social skills to help them increase their interaction with each other as well as their classroom peers.

Referral: These children were referred to an occupational therapy group situation for evaluation and treatment of their psychosocial interpersonal skills.

Progress Report: Initially each child demanded excessive personal attention. Sharing and cooperation skills were weak. Their frustration level was high, their attention span was short, and they showed general inability to problem-solve. Two of the children have limited communication skills, which sometimes lead to hitting or shouting. As of this date, the group has been together for 1 month. They have made some progress in using the phrases of "please, thank you, and please pass—" instead of grabbing from each other. They are now able to sit in a circle and pass items quietly from left to right. They are able to follow simple two-step directions without demonstrating frustration.

2. Intervention Goals

a. Long-Term Goals

The long-term goal for each of these children is to be able to interact in groups, with peers, and with other people in various social settings.

b. Short-Term Goals

The short-term goal is for the children to complete a simple group activity of their choosing that demonstrates the progress that they are making in working together.

3. Goal-Directed Purposeful Activity Description

The Parent-Teachers Association of School #27 is sponsoring a bake sale next Tuesday and all the classes are invited to participate. The practitioner and children discussed the possibility of baking cookies together, and the group voted to make chocolate chip cookies from a recipe and to use all fresh ingredients.

4. Activity Preparation

a. Review Goals, Describe Practitioner's Role

In view of the goals for increased group interaction and cooperation, the occupational therapist will choose a chocolate chip cookie recipe and determine how each child can participate. The practitioner will shop for the ingredients. The practitioner will visit the school kitchen supervisor to request permission to use space in the kitchen for 1 hour and 15 minutes. Together they will select the baking equipment the children will use. The practitioner will request the help of an aide from the kitchen staff to assist with the treatment session. The practitioner will also request permission to walk the children through the kitchen prior to the treatment session to acquaint them with its sights and sounds.

b. Personnel Required to Do the Preparation

One practitioner.

c. Required Preparation Time

Approximately 1½ hours.

d. Required Place and Space
Grocery store to shop for the ingredients. Refrigerator space for ingredients.

e. Materials
n/a

f. Equipment
Car to drive to the grocery store.

g. Safety Precautions for Personnel
None required.

5. Activity Implementation
   a. Personnel
   Practitioner, the children, and one school aide.

   b. Setting and Location
   The activity will take place in the school kitchen during the mid-afternoon when the kitchen is not in use.

   c. Space Required
   Space is needed for two cafeteria tables and six chairs. Five children and two adults need to be able to move around the tables easily. The surrounding space needs to be arranged to limit the children's movement and attention to the table activity. Wheelchair space at the table is required.

   d. Environment
   The environment should be as calming as possible. This will be a challenge in a school kitchen with all the stainless steel workspace and appliances. Covering the children's workspace with clean bath towels will help dampen the noise and prevent utensils from sliding. The practitioner and aide will use quiet voices and tones as they direct the children. It would be wise to take the children through the kitchen prior to their cookie baking day to acquaint them with the sights and sounds.

   e. Materials
   Cookie ingredients, shortening for the cookie sheets, paper towels to wipe up spills and sticky fingers, napkins and juice to enjoy with finished cookies, and a large plastic trash bag.

   f. Equipment: Assistive Devices and Adaptations Included
   Small equipment includes a medium-size non-breakable mixing bowl, a small electric mixer, mixing spoons, measuring cups and spoons, metal spatula, two cookie sheets, two cooling racks, a small basket for serving cookies, a large plastic container for storing the finished cookies, a cookie timer, and bath towels to cover the tables. Two six-person tables and four chairs will be brought from the cafeteria. One will be the children's work table and the other will hold the supplies. The kitchen oven is near the workspace.

   g. Required Intervention Time
   One hour for the activity and 15 minutes for cleanup.

   h. Safety Precautions for Client
   Because all of the children have patterns of unpredictable behavior, they must be monitored closely to keep them on activity. The practitioner and aide must closely supervise the children as they use the materials and equipment.

6. Client-Practitioner Activity Sequence (10 action steps or less)
   1. *While the practitioner is positioning the children around the work table, the aide will measure each of the ingredients into small bowls that the children can carry and place on the supply table. The mixing bowl and mixing spoon will be placed on the work table.*

2. *The practitioner will read the list of ingredients, then direct or assist each child to go to the supply table to pick up the bowl containing the assigned ingredient and return to the table. The aide will assist the child in choosing the correct bowl if necessary.*

3. *When the children are seated, the mixing bowl will be passed from left to right and each child will add an ingredient to the bowl.*

4. *The mixing bowl will be passed a second time and each child will have a turn at mixing the contents with a mixing spoon. Both the practitioner and the aide will assist as necessary. The aide will do the final mixing with a hand mixer.*

5. *As the bowl is passed again, each child will place a spoonful of cookie dough on a prepared cookie sheet.*

6. *The aide will place the filled cookie sheets in the preheated oven. The timer will be set on the table where the children can watch it.*

7. *While the aide supervises the baking, the practitioner and the children will talk about the cookie baking process and how each child participated. The practitioner will point out the positive aspects of their behavior while working together. The children will be encouraged to talk about their feelings.*

8. *When the timer rings, the aide will remove the cookies from the oven and place them on cooling racks. Seven cookies will be placed in a small basket.*

9. *The children will pass the cookie basket around the circle from left to right and enjoy a treat. The children will share their cookies with the aide and practitioner. Juice and a napkin will be passed to each child.*

10. *Everyone will help clean up the work site and the cooled cookies will be placed in a covered plastic container ready to go to the bake sale. The practitioner and the children will thank the aide for helping them.*

7. Uniform Terminology Documentation
    I. Performance Areas
        A. Activities of Daily Living
            10. Socialization
            11. Functional Communication
    II. Performance Components
        C. Psychosocial Skills and Psychological Components
            2. Social
                a. Role Performance
                b. Social Conduct
                c. Interpersonal Skills
            3. Self-Management
                a. Coping Skills
                c. Self-Control
    III. Performance Contexts
        A. Temporal Aspects
            1. Chronological
            2. Developmental
            4. Disability Status

NOTES

NOTES

NOTES

Unit Nine

Utilizing Assistive Technology
The Forms Website

Your book has been provided with a colored insert (located inside the front cover) that contains your individual password to use the *Activity Analysis & Application, Fourth Edition* Online Forms Download Website, located on the Internet at:

http://www.slackbooks.com/forms/

Here you may download blank copies of the following forms free of charge:

- ❖ Activity Awareness Form
- ❖ Action Identification Form
- ❖ Activity Analysis for Expected Performance
- ❖ Activity Analysis for Therapeutic Intervention
- ❖ Client-Activity Correlation Form

These forms can only be downloaded one time, so please be sure to read the saving instructions that appear on the website carefully before proceeding to download them. The forms must be saved either onto a disk or onto your computer's hard drive.

Important: After downloading, your password will be void.

The five forms are for your personal use in the classroom, for practice, or in an evaluation setting.

If you encounter any problems in downloading your *Activity Analysis & Application, Fourth Edition* forms, please email SLACK Incorporated's Technical Support at *Techsupport@slackinc.com* or call 856-848-2186 Monday through Friday 9:00 am to 5:00 pm, Eastern Standard Time.

EPILOGUE

There is a story tradition that carries remarkable impact for occupational therapy practitioners. Two fishermen were fly casting in a stream when they noticed with dismay a group of children floating down the river. Some of the children were struggling to remain above the water, others were floundering unsuccessfully, a few were managing to make it ashore unaided. The men abandoned their poles to help rescue the children, but more and more continued to come down the river. Suddenly, one of the fishermen rushed to the shore and started running upstream along the bank. The other called out to him not to leave because he could not manage to save the children alone. The departing fisherman yelled back, "Save those you can. I'm going to stop the person who's pushing them in" (West, 1973, p. 19). This story bears an analogy to the community and was given originally to introduce a range of issues facing health professionals. But it also suggests some remarkable parallels to what the student has experienced in using this text. Analyzing what activity was needed in the situation dictated the occupational performance needs of both fishermen. The meaning and purpose of their occupation changed when a further aspect of the problem surfaced in the mind of one fisherman. The steps to make real intervention is revealed in the drastic decision to leave the other fisherman.

This handbook has been presented as a framework for thinking about activity in all its dimensions. Learning the process of activity analysis is a basic skill that all occupational therapy students must have before applying it toward an intervention model. The authors have offered the student a beginning level of knowledge in how activities can be used in intervention and relate to specific goals of a given client. "To use purposeful activity therapeutically, (a practitioner) analyzes the activity from several perspectives. ...All this information is considered together to assist... in synthesizing (i.e., adapting, grading, and combining) activities for therapeutic purposes for a particular individual" (American Occupational Therapy Association, 1993). Purposeful activity is the medium of occupational therapy, and activity analysis serves as a baseline for understanding the importance of this concept.

Using Uniform Terminology as the language to translate each activity into a treatment modality has proven to be a positive tool for understanding the dimensions of activity. Through all its revisions, and now entering another, Uniform Terminology has provided a structure for communicating in words how activity is used in intervention. Because it exists outside the boundaries of any particular frame of reference, Uniform Terminology can serve as a neutral means of conveying information about the client and the output of therapeutic intervention. It continues to perform the job of providing a uniform description base for the profession.

The authors have collaborated to create a template for students with which they might grasp the basic concepts of activity analysis. This has been an evolutionary process taking place over the past 17 years and has led across confronting detours, diverse paths of thinking, and many avenues of debate. The end of the road has not been reached. This textbook is only an introduction in the clinical reasoning process. With experience and practice, this kind of analysis will become an automatic thinking pattern. "Activity analysis and syntheses [Mosey, 1986] are then used to design therapeutic occupations to remediate the person's impairments that are limiting occupational performance" (Fisher, 1998, p. 519). Skills and abilities in clinical reasoning will grow through increasing contact with clients in delivering occupational therapy intervention. No one textbook, class, or professional degree fulfills the need for life-long learning. Education in this area will come through formal and informal learning situations, from continuing education workshops and conferences, from colleagues, professional literature, and, most of all, from clients.

Activity analysis and its application will remain one of the practitioner's most valuable assets in the future. As a profession, our potential has only begun to be realized. Returning to the basic beliefs in the power of occupation and purposeful activity has given added momentum to reach out to the community and reveal possibilities not dreamed of before. The writings of the recipients of the Eleanor Clarke Slagle Lectureship provide direction for the future of the profession. A striking aspect of these articles is the discrepancy between the findings of research and the limited scope of today's practice. Untapped population-based groups have needs that occupation-based intervention can fulfill. Areas such as the rise in the aging population, the focus on ergonomics, the assistive technology revolution, prevention practice arenas, the focus on addressing spirituality issues, and the constant change in medical treatment approaches are part of this potential. There are segments of the population of every community that are failing to realize the potential standards of health possible. The continued rate of abuse of drugs, chemicals, children, and spouses; the high rate of divorce, suicide and violent crime; the presence of malnutrition, poverty, pollution and unsatisfactory employment, all point to a pathology from which no community is immune (Gross & Moyer, 1977, p. 2). The health of the community is undeniably bound up with the health of the individuals residing in it (Rosenfeld, 1982, p. 235). A responsibility to address such areas is crucial, and practitioners must broaden their horizons to develop the many facets of that professional base called occupation. The challenge as a profession is to open the door to a wider view of how purposeful activity makes life worth living.

One way to meet this challenge is teaching the occupational therapy student the art and skill of making activity meaningful and purposeful. Further study in theory, frames of reference, treatment modalities, medical problems, and disabling conditions must be supplemented with problems facing the well population, health prevention, quality of life, and alleviation of barriers limiting the ability to function independently. Working from a knowledge founded on the intimate relationship between actively doing and health, the occupational therapy practitioner believes in the intrinsic value of goal-directed activity to attain a purpose in life and a sense of well-being (Sorensen, 1978, p. 288). Exploring and reflecting on the research and philosophy of such terms as occupation, purposeful activity, function, independence, and health results in a solid background and confidence to move forward into new practice arenas. The leadership of those from the past combined with the personal strengths and capabilities of today's practitioners will bring the profession into a strong tomorrow. As shown in the opening story, a difference in perspective can be the key.

REFERENCES

American Occupational Therapy Association (1993). Position paper: Purposeful activity. *American Journal of Occupational Therapy, 47*, 1081-1082.

Fisher, A. G. (1998). Uniting practice and theory in an occupational framework: 1998 Eleanor Clarke Slagle Lecture. *American Journal of Occupational Therapy, 52*(7).

Gross, D. M., & Moyer, E. A. (1977). *Occupational therapy in the community.* New York: New York State OT Association, Inc.

Rosenfeld, M. S. (1982). A model for activity intervention in disaster-stricken communities. *American Journal of Occupational Therapy, 36*(4).

Sorensen, J. (1978). Occupational therapy in business: A new horizon. *American Journal of Occupational Therapy, 32*(5).

West, W. (1973). The growing importance of prevention. In L. A. Llorens (Ed.), *Consultation in the community: Occupational therapy in child health.* Dubuque, Iowa: Kendall/Hunt.

NOTES

NOTES

NOTES

SUGGESTED READING

Adelstein, L. A., & Nelson, D. L. (1985). Effects of sharing versus nonsharing on affective meaning in collage activities. *Occupational Therapy in Mental Health, 5,* 29-45.

Allen, C. (1982). Independence through activity: The practice of occupational therapy (psychiatry). *American Journal of Occupational Therapy, 36,* 731-739.

Allen, C. K. (1985). *OT for psychiatric diseases: Measurement and management of cognitive disabilities.* Boston, MA: Little, Brown & Co.

Allen, C. K., Earnart, C. A., & Blue, T. (1992). *Occupational therapy treatment goals for the physically and cognitively disabled.* Rockville, MD: AOTA.

AOTA Commission on Practice. (1998). Position paper: The use of general information and assistive technology within occupational therapy. *American Journal of Occupational Therapy, 52* (10), 870-71.

Bakshi, R., Bhambhani, Y., & Madill, H. (1991). The effects of task preference on performance during purposeful and nonpurposeful activities. *American Journal of Occupational Therapy, 45,* 912-916.

Banning, M. R., & Nelson, D. L. (1987). The effects of activity-elicited humor and group structure on group cohesion and affective meanings. *American Journal of Occupational Therapy, 41,* 510-514.

Baum, C. & Law, M. (1997). Occupational therapy practice: Focusing on occupational performance. *American Journal of Occupational Therapy, 51,* 277-288.

Bissell, J., & Mailloux, Z. (1981). The use of crafts in occupational therapy for the physically disabled. *American Journal of Occupational Therapy, 35,* 369-374.

Bloch, M., Smith, D., & Nelson, D. (1989). Heart rate, activity, duration, and affect in added-purpose versus single-purpose jumping activities. *American Journal of Occupational Therapy, 43,* 25-29.

Borst, & Nelson, D. L. (1993). Use of uniform terminology by occupational therapy students. *American Journal of Occupational Therapy, 47,* 611.

Breines, E. (2000). In times of bereavement. *Advance for Occupational Therapy Practitioners, March 13, 25.*

Breines, E. B. (1995). *Occupational therapy activities from clay to computers, theory and practice.* Philadelphia, PA: F. A. Davis Co.

Bundy, A. C. (1993). Assessment of play and leisure: Delineation of the problem. *American Journal of Occupational Therapy, 47* (3), 217-222.

Carter, B. A., Nelson, D. L., & Duncombe, L. W. (1983). The effect of psychological type on the mood and meaning of two collage activities. *American Journal of Occupational Therapy, 39,* 688-693.

Chandani, A., & Hill, C. (1990). What really is therapeutic activity? *British Journal of Occupational Therapy, 53,* 15-18.

Christiansen, C., & Baum, C. (1991). *Occupational therapy: Overcoming human performance deficits.* Thorofare, NJ: SLACK Incorporated.

Clark, P. N. (1979). Human development through occupation: Theoretical frameworks in contemporary occupational therapy practice. *American Journal of Occupational Therapy, 33,* 505-514.

Cottrell, R. P. F. (1996). *Perspectives on purposeful activity: Foundation and future of occupational therapy.* Bethesda, MD: AOTA.

Crabtree, J. (1998). The end of occupational therapy. *American Journal of Occupational Therapy, 52,* 205-214.

Crepeau, E. B. (1998). Activity analysis: A way of thinking about occupational performance. In M. E. Neistadt & E. B. Crepeau (Eds.), *Willard & Spackman's occupational therapy, 9th Ed.* pp. (135-147).

DiJoseph, L. (1982). Independence through activity: Mind, body, and environment interaction in therapy. *American Journal of Occupational Therapy, 36,* 740-744.

Drake, M. (1992). *Crafts in therapy and rehabilitation.* Thorofare, NJ: SLACK Incorporated.

Drake, M. (1999). *Crafts in therapy and rehabilitation, 2nd Ed.* Thorofare, NJ: SLACK Incorporated.

Dunn, W. (1982). Independence through activity: The practice of occupational therapy (pediatrics). *American Journal of Occupational Therapy, 36,* 745-747.

Dunn, W., Brown, C., & McGuigan, A. (1994). The ecology of human performance: A framework for considering the effect of context. *American Journal of Occupational Therapy, 48(7),* 595-607.

Dunn, W., & McGourty, L. (1989). Application of uniform terminology to practice. *American Journal of Occupational Therapy, 43,* 817-831.

Dunton, W. R. Jr. (1923). A debate upon toy-making as a therapeutic occupation: Con. *Archives of Occupational Therapy, 2,* 39-43.

Dunton, W. R. Jr. (1923). Rejoiner. *Archives of Occupational Therapy, 2,* 47.

Fahl, M. A. (1970). Emotionally disturbed children: Effects of cooperative and competitive activity on peer interaction. *American Journal of Occupational Therapy, 24,* 31-33.

Fidler, G. S. (1948). Psychological evaluation of occupational therapy activities. *American Journal of Occupational Therapy, 2,* 284-287.

Fidler, G. S. (1969). The task-oriented group as a context for treatment. *American Journal of Occupational Therapy, 23,* 43-48.

Fidler, G. S. (1981). From crafts to competence. *American Journal of Occupational Therapy, 35,* 567-573.

Fidler, G. S. (1996). Life-style performance: From profile to conceptual model. *American Journal of Occupational Therapy, 50 (2),* 139-147.

Fidler, G. S., & Fidler, J. W. (1978). Doing and becoming: Purposeful action and self-actualization. *American Journal of Occupational Therapy, 32,* 305-310.

Fitts, H. A., & Howe, M. C. (1987). Use of leisure time by cardiac patients. *American Journal of Occupational Therapy, 41,* 583-589.

Fox, J., & Jirgal, D. (1967). Therapeutic properties of activities as examined by the clinical council of the Wisconsin schools of O.T. *American Journal of Occupational Therapy, 21,* 29-33.

Froehlich, J., & Nelson, D. L. (1986). Affective meanings of life review through activities and discussion. *American Journal of Occupational Therapy, 40,* 27-33.

Gliner, J. A. (1985). Purposeful activity in motor learning theory: An event approach to motor skill acquisition. *American Journal of Occupational Therapy, 39,* 28-34.

Grady, A. P. (1992). Occupation as vision. *American Journal of Occupational Therapy, 46 (12),* 1062-1065.

Haase, B. (1995). Clinical interpretation of "occupationally embedded exercise versus rote exercise: A choice between occupational forms by elderly nursing home residents." *American Journal of Occupational Therapy, 49,* 403-404.

Hatter, J. K., & Nelson, D. L. (1987). Altruism and task participation in the elderly. *American Journal of Occupational Therapy, 41,* 379-381.

Henry, A. D., Nelson, D. L., & Duncombe, L. W. (1984). Choice-making in group and individual activity. *American Journal of Occupational Therapy, 38,* 245-251.

Hoover, J. A. B. (1996). Diversional occupational therapy in World War I: A need for purpose in occupations. *American Journal of Occupational Therapy, 50*(10),881-885.

Howard, B. S. & J. R. (1997). Occupation as spiritual activity. *American Journal of Occupational Therapy, 51* (3), 181-185.

Huss, J. (1981). From kinesiology to adaptation. *American Journal of Occupational Therapy, 35,* 574-580.

Jacobshagen, I. (1990). The effect of interruption of activity of affect. *Occupational Therapy in Mental Health, 10*(2), 35-46.

Jongbloed, L., & Morgan, D. (1991). An investigation of involvement in leisure activities after a stroke. *American Journal of Occupational Therapy, 45,* 420-427.

Katz, N., & Cohen, E. (1991). Meanings ascribed to four craft activities before and after extensive learning. *Occupational Therapy Journal of Research, 11*(1), 24-39.

Kielhofner, G. (1980). A model of human occupation, Part 2. Ontogenesis perspective of temporal adaptation. *American Journal of Occupational Therapy, 34,* 657-663.

Kielhofner, G. (1980). A model of human occupation, Part 3. Benign and vicious cycles. *American Journal of Occupational Therapy, 34,* 731-737.

Kielhofner, G. (1982). A heritage of activity: Development of theory. *American Journal of Occupational Therapy, 36,* 723-730.

Kielhofner, G., & Burke, J. P. (1980). A model of human occupation, Part 1. Conceptual framework and content. *American Journal of Occupational Therapy, 34,* 572-581.

Kielhofner, G., Burke, J. P., & Igi, C. H. (1980). A model of human occupation, Part 4. Assessment and intervention. *American Journal of Occupational Therapy, 34,* 777-788.

Kircher, M. A. (1984). Motivation as a factor of perceived exertion in purposeful versus nonpurposeful activity. *American Journal of Occupational Therapy, 38,* 165-170.

Kleinman, B. L., & Stalcup, A. (1991). The effect of a graded craft activities on visuomotor integration in an inpatient child psychiatry population. *American Journal of Occupational Therapy, 45,* 324-330.

Kremer, E. R. H., Nelson, D. L., & Duncombe, L. W. (1984). Effects of selected activities on affective meaning in psychiatric clients. *American Journal of Occupational Therapy, 38,* 522-528.

Lang, E., Nelson, D., & Bush, M. (1992). Comparison of performance in materials-based occupation, imagery-based occupation, and rote exercise in nursing home residents. *American Journal of Occupational Therapy, 46,* 607-611.

Lerner, C. J. (1979). The magazine picture collage. *American Journal of Occupational Therapy, 33*(8), 500-504.

Levine, R. E., & Brayley, C. R. (1991). Occupation as a therapeutic medium: A contextual approach to performance intervention. In C. Christiansen, & C. Baum (Eds.), *Occupational therapy: Overcoming human performance deficits* (pp. 590-631). Thorofare, NJ: SLACK Incorporated.

Llorens, L. A. (1986). Activity analysis: Agreement among factors in a sensory processing model. *American Journal of Occupational Therapy, 40,* 103-110.

Lyon, B. G. (1983). Purposeful versus human activity. *American Journal of Occupational Therapy, 37,* 493-495.

Miller, L., & Nelson, D. L. (1987). Dual-purpose activity versus single-purpose activity in terms of duration on task, exertion level, and affect. *Occupational Therapy in Mental Health, 7,* 55-67.

Mullins, C. S., Nelson, D. L., & Smith, D. A. (1987). Exercise through dual-purpose activity in the institutionalized elderly. *Physical and Occupational Therapy in Geriatrics, 5,* 29-39.

Mumford, M. (1974). A comparison of interpersonal skills in verbal and activity groups. *American Journal of Occupational Therapy, 28,* 281-283.

Nelson, D. L. (1988). Occupation: Form and performance. *American Journal of Occupational Therapy, 42,* 633-641.

Nelson, D. L. (1996). Therapeutic occupation: A definition. *American Journal of Occupational Therapy, 50*(10), 775-782.

Nelson, D. L., & Peterson C. (1989). Enhancing therapeutic exercise through purposeful activity: A theoretic analysis. *Topics in Geriatric Rehabilitation, 4*(4), 12-22.

Nelson, D. L., Peterson C., Smith D. A., Boughton J. A., & Whalen G. M. (1988). Effects of project versus parallel groups on social interaction and affective responses in senior citizens. *American Journal of Occupational Therapy, 42*, 23-29.

Nelson, D. L., Thompson G., & Moore J. A. (1982). Identification of factors of affective meaning in four selected activities. *American Journal of Occupational Therapy, 36*, 381-387.

Niswander, P., & Hyde R. (1954). The value of crafts in psychiatric occupational therapy. *American Journal of Occupational Therapy, 8*, 104-106.

Peloquin, S. M. (1991). Occupational therapy service: Individual and collective understandings of the founders, Part 2. *American Journal of Occupational Therapy, 45*, 733-744.

Petrone, P. (1994). Clinical interpretation of "the relationship between occupational form and occupational performance: A kinematic perspective." *American Journal of Occupational Therapy, 48*, 688.

Pianetti, C., Palacios, M., & Elliott, L. (1964). Significance of color. *American Journal of Occupational Therapy, 18*, 137-140.

Polatajko, H. (1994). Dreams, dilemmas, and decisions for occupational therapy in the new millennium: A Canadian perspective. *American Journal of Occupational Therapy, 48*, 590-594.

Quiroga, V. A. M. (1995). *Occupational therapy: The first 30 years, 1900 to 1930.* Rockville, MD: AOTA.

Rocker, J. D., & Nelson, D. L. (1987). Affective responses to keeping and not keeping an activity product. *American Journal of Occupational Therapy, 41*, 152-157.

Rothaus, P., Hanson, P., & Cleveland, S. (1966). Art and group dynamics. *American Journal of Occupational Therapy, 20*, 182-187.

Royeen, C. B., Cynkin, S., & Robinson, A. M. (1990). Analyzing performance through activity. *AOTA Self Study Series: Assessing Function, No. 5.* Rockville, MD: AOTA.

Scardina, V. (1981). From pegboards to integration. *American Journal of Occupational Therapy, 35*, 581-588.

Schemm, R. (1994). Looking back: Bridging conflicting ideologies. The origins of American and British occupational therapy. *American Journal of Occupational Therapy, 48*, 1082-1087.

Shing-Ru Shih, L., Nelson, D. L., & Duncombe, L. W. (1984). Mood and affect following success and failure in two cultural groups. *Occupational Therapy Journal of Research, 4*, 213-230.

Shontz, F. C. (1959). Evaluation of psychological effects. *American Journal of Physical Medicine, 38*, 138-142.

Simon, C. J. (1993). Use of activity and activity analysis. In H. L. Hopkins, & H. D. Smith (Eds.), *Willard & Spackman's occupational therapy, 8th Ed.* (pp. 281-292). Philadelphia, PA: J. B. Lippincott Co.

Slade, S., Falkowski, W., Muwonge, A. K., & Slade, P. (1975). Immediate psychological effects of various occupational therapy activities on psychiatric patients: A pilot study. *British Journal of Occupational Therapy, 38*, 172-173.

Smith, P. A., Barrows, H. S., & Whitney, J. N. (1959). Psychological attributes of occupational therapy crafts. *American Journal of Occupational Therapy, 13*, 16-21, 25-26.

Steffan, J. A., & Nelson, D. L. (1987). The effects of tool scarcity on group climate and affective meaning within the context of a stenciling activity. *American Journal of Occupational Therapy, 41*, 449-453.

Steinbeck, T. M. (1986). Purposeful activity and performance. *American Journal of Occupational Therapy, 40*, 529-534.

Taber, F., Baron, S., & Blackwell, A. (1953). A study of a task directed and a free choice group. *American Journal of Occupational Therapy, 7*, 118-124.

Taylor, E., & Manguno, J. (1990). Use of treatment activities in occupational therapy. *American Journal of Occupational Therapy, 45*(4), 317-322.

Thibodeaux, D., & Ludwig, F. (1988). Intrinsic motivation in product-oriented and non-product-oriented activities. *American Journal of Occupational Therapy, 42*, 169-175.

Watson, D. E. (1997). *Task analysis: An occupational performance approach.* Bethesda, MD: AOTA.

Weston, D. L. (1960). Therapeutic crafts. *American Journal of Occupational Therapy, 14,* 121-123.

Weston, D. L. (1961). The dimensions of crafts. *American Journal of Occupational Therapy, 15,* 1-5.

Williamson, G. G. (1982). The heritage of activity: Development of theory. *American Journal of Occupational Therapy, 36,* 716-722.

Wood, W. (1995). Weaving the warp and weft of occupational therapy: An art and science for all times. *American Journal of Occupational Therapy, 49,* 44-52.

Wu, C., Trombly, C., & Lin, K. (1994). The relationship between occupational form and occupational performance: A kinematic perspective. *American Journal of Occupational Therapy, 48,* 679-687.

Yerxa, E. (1994). Dreams, dilemmas, and decisions for occupational therapy in the new millennium: An American perspective. *American Journal of Occupational Therapy, 48,* 586-589.

Yoder, R. M., Nelson, D. L., & Smith, D. A. (1989). Added-purpose versus rote exercise in female nursing home residents. *American Journal of Occupational Therapy, 43,* 581-586.

Zimmerer-Branum, S., & Nelson, D. (1995). Occupationally embedded exercise versus rote exercise: A choice between occupational forms by elderly nursing home residents. *American Journal of Occupational Therapy, 49,* 397-404.

APPENDICES

Appendix A

AMERICAN OCCUPATIONAL THERAPY ASSOCIATION
POSITION PAPERS

POSITION PAPER: OCCUPATION

Concern with the occupational nature of human beings was fundamental to the establishment of occupational therapy. Since the time of occupational therapy's founding, the term *occupation* has been used to refer to an individual's active participation in self-maintenance, work, leisure, and play (American Occupational Therapy Association [AOTA], 1993; Bing, 1981; Levine, 1991; Meyer, 1922). Within the literature of the field, however, the meaning of occupation has been ambiguous because the term has been used interchangeably with other concepts. This paper's intent is to distinguish the term *occupation* from other terms, to summarize traditional beliefs about its nature and therapeutic value, and to identify factors that have impeded the study and discussion of occupation.

The Dynamic, Multidimensional Nature of Occupations

Occupations are the normal and familiar things that people do every day. This simple description reflects, but understates, the multidimensional and complex nature of daily occupation.

Occupations can be broadly explained as having both performance and contextual dimensions because they involve acts within defined settings (Christiansen, 1991; Nelson, 1988; Rogers, 1982). In that they frequently extend over time, occupations have a temporal dimension (Kielhofner, 1977; Meyer, 1922). Further, in that engagement in occupation is seen to be driven by an intrinsic need for mastery, competence, self-identity, and group acceptance, occupations have a psychological dimension (Brown, 1986; Burke, 19--; Christiansen, 1994; DiMatteo, 1991; Fidler & Fidler, 1979, 1983; White, 1971). Since occupations are often associated with a social or occupational role and are therefore identifiable in the culture, they have social and symbolic dimensions (Mosey, 1986; Fidler & Fidler, 1983; Frank, 1994). Finally, because they are infused with meaning within the lives of individuals, occupations have spiritual dimensions (Clark, 1993; Mattingly & Fleming, 1993). The term *spiritual* is used here to refer to the nonphysical and nonmaterial aspects of existence. In this sense, it is postulated that daily pursuits contribute insight into the nature and meaning of a person's life.

This multidimensional view of occupations and their central place in the experience of living was recognized early in the profession's history. Influenced by the pragmatic philosophies of John Dewey and William James (Breines, 1987), which related well-being to an individual's participation in the world around him or her, early theorists such as Tracy (1910), Dunton (1918), and Slagle (1922) contended that doing things favorably influenced interest and attention, provided relaxation, promoted moral development, reenergized the individual, normalized habits, and conferred a physical benefit (Upham, 1918).

Adolph Meyer (1922) asserted that, for healthy people, daily living unfolds in a natural and balanced pattern of occupational pursuits that bring both satisfaction and fulfillment. He noted that occupations have a performance or doing component, as well as a spiritual or personal meaning component. Meyer recognized that through daily occupations, people organized their lives in terms of time and made meaning of their existence as human beings. Meyer believed that the organizing, self-fulfilling characteristics of occupations could make them an important mechanism of adaptation. He postulated that the individual could affect his or her state of health through occupations selected and performed each day. This view has been a principle of many conceptual frames of reference developed by occupational therapy scholars since that time (Christiansen, 1991; Kielhofner, 1993; Reilly, 1962).

In summary, occupational therapy scholars agree that human occupations have emotional, cognitive, physical, spiritual, and contextual dimensions, all of which are related to general well-being. However, occupational therapy scholars have not been able to agree on the specific concepts regarding these dimensions, or on specific terms to name them.

Distinguishing Between Occupation and Related Terms

The physical and mental abilities and skills required for satisfactory engagement in a given occupational pursuit constitute the performance dimension of human occupation, often referred to in the occupational therapy literature as *occupational performance*. The performance dimension of occupations is that aspect which has received the most study and attention in the history of the field. This may explain why the terms *function* and *purposeful activity* have been used as synonyms for engagement in occupation (Henderson et al., 1991).

Occupations, because of their intentional nature, always involve mental abilities and skills, and typically, but not always, have an observable physical or active dimension. Whether one is laying bricks or practicing meditation exercises, one can be said to be "doing" something. Only one of these occupations, however, requires observable physical action. Whether physical or mental in nature, the behaviors necessary for completion of tasks in daily occupations can be analyzed according to specific com-

ponents related to moving, perceiving, thinking, and feeling. Various occupational performance components have been described and defined within the *Uniform Terminology for Occupational Therapy, Third Edition* (AOTA, 1994).

Position papers on function and purposeful activity have been developed by the AOTA, and it is important to clarify the differences in meaning between these terms and the term *occupation*. The AOTA has proposed that when occupational therapists use the term *function*, they refer to an individual's *performance* of activities, tasks, and roles during daily occupations (occupational performance) (AOTA, 1995). Purposeful activity has also been recognized as a term to describe engagement in the tasks of daily living, with the use of this term emphasizing the intentional, goal directed nature of such engagement (AOTA, 1993). In this paper, it is proposed that reference to human occupation necessarily encompasses the required human capacities to act on the environment with intentionality in a given pursuit, as well as the unique organization of these pursuits over time and the meanings attributed to them by doers as well as those observing them.

In summary, occupations have performance, contextual, temporal, psychological, social, symbolic, and spiritual dimensions; whereas function in its specific use denotes primarily the performance dimension. While the term *purposeful activity* recognizes multiple dimensions and emphasizes intentionality, it is viewed as a term that does not capture the richness of human enterprise embodied in the word *occupation*. It is asserted that while all occupations constitute purposeful activity, not all purposeful activities can be described as occupations.

Therapeutic Benefits of Occupations

Since Adolph Meyer's (1922) philosophical essay, many scholarly papers have been written about the therapeutic value of occupations (Clark, 1993; Cynkin & Robinson, 1990; Englehardt, 1977; Reilly, 1962; Yerxa, 1967). These have identified a broad scope of benefits, ranging from the facilitation of habilitation, adaptation, and self-actualization to improvements in motor control and sensory processing. While there is growing evidence to support some of these claims, additional research is needed before it can be demonstrated that other benefits are likely valid.

Because occupation is an extremely complex phenomenon and has not been subjected to rigorous research until recently, many questions about its nature and its relationship to health and well-being remain unanswered. This emphasizes the need for further study. Current beliefs and theories about occupation should be regarded as incomplete and evolving.

Forces Advancing and Impeding the Study and Discussion of Occupation

One of the problems inhibiting the study of occupations is how to clearly, logically, and consistently describe different levels and types of occupations. Used here, the term *levels* refers to the complexity of a given occupation. For example, while getting dressed and driving to work are readily interpretable as organized sets of actions that may partially comprise a typical day, each of these involves a variety of specific and definable behaviors, such as buttoning a shirt or turning an ignition key, which are less complex. Even occupational behaviors of greater complexity, such as dressing or driving, are nested within clusters of activity that comprise and are recognized as part of larger sets of organized behavior within cultures, such as pursuing a career. This phenomenon of nesting, where simple acts can be identified as parts of more complex sets of acts, is a dimension of occupations that relates to their organization over time and can be viewed as reflecting varying levels of complexity.

The English language has words associated with occupations, such as *actions*, *tasks*, and *projects*, which imply differences in complexity. Evans (1987) and Kielhofner (1993) have been among those who have described the hierarchical nature of occupations, and others (Christiansen, 1991; Nelson, 1988) have suggested that it would be useful if specific terms for human enterprise denoted different levels of this hierarchy. However, there is little agreement among scholars in occupational therapy or in the social sciences for how these terms ought to be used to describe varying levels of complexity in occupational behavior.

Similar difficulties exist in describing types or categories of occupations. Certain categories of occupations have gained conventional usage by occupational therapists and are recognized in contemporary culture. These include work, self-care (or maintenance), play, and leisure.

Studies of human beings in different cultures have shown similarities in time use according to these general categories (Christiansen, in press). However, while general categories of occupations are recognized across cultures, the specific tasks that constitute each category and the delineation of categories vary across individuals. The classification of a given task within a larger category seems to be dependent upon the context in which it is performed. For example, sewing may be viewed as work by some and classified as leisure by others.

Similarly, most occupational pursuits seem to have both a general or cultural meaning attributed by participants and observers as well as a specific and personal meaning known only to the performer (Nelson, 1988; Rommerveit, 1980). Consider, for example, that getting dressed is viewed as a necessary and practical aspect of daily life in most cultures, but assumes symbolic importance when it is performed without assistance for the first time by the 3-year-old child, or by an adult mastering use of a new prosthetic arm. Dressing in anticipation of a ceremony or developmental milestone, such as high school graduation or a wedding, imbues the act with special significance. Over time, the experiences embedded in daily occupations assume collective meaning and are interpreted as essential part of a person's self- narrative or life story (Bruner, 1990; Clark, 1993; Mattingly & Fleming, 1993).

Research on Occupations and Research in Occupational Therapy

It is useful to recognize that research on occupations should be distinguished from research in occupational therapy (Mosey, 1992). In the first instance, inquiry is directed toward understanding the nature of the typical daily occupations in which people engage; that is, what people do, how they do it, and why they do it. The study of occupational therapy, conversely, concerns itself with the effect of occupation on health, development of frames of reference that facilitate the identification and remediation of occupational dysfunction, and other topical issues of significance to this science-based profession.

Research for both areas has been impeded by the lack of conventional definitions for terms related to occupation. This, in turn, has contributed to disagreements about the proper concern of practice and the appropriate focus of research (Christiansen, 1981, 1991; Kielhofner & Burke, 1997; Mosey, 1985, 1989; Rogers, 1982; Shannon, 1977). Recently, occupational science has emerged as an area of study concerned with understanding humans as occupational beings (Clark, et al., 1991; Yerxa, et al., 1989). As additional research enables us to learn more about the nature of occupations and their potential as a means for promoting and restoring health and well-being, it is likely that there will be continued discussion on the use of terminology to describe specific concepts.

This paper has attempted to identify distinctions among current terms related to human occupation. As our understanding of occupations advances, more concepts and terms will evolve. It is important to continue to develop knowledge about occupations to facilitate our further understanding of an important, complex, and rich aspect of human life. In this way, the profession of occupational therapy will better appreciate the vision of its founders, more clearly understand its current state, and more likely realize the potential embodied in occupations as touchstones of human existence.

References

American Occupational Therapy Association. (1993). Position paper: Purposeful Activity. American *Journal of Occupational Therapy, 47,* 1081-1082.

American Occupational Therapy Association. (1994). Uniform terminology for occupational therapy - Third edition. *American Journal of Occupational Therapy, 48,* 1047-1059.

American Occupational Therapy Association. (1995). Position paper: Occupational performance: Occupational therapy's definition of function. *American Journal of Occupational Therapy, 49,* 1019-1020.

Bing, R. (1981). Occupational therapy revisited: A paraphrastic journey. *American Journal of Occupational Therapy, 35,* 499-518.

Breines, E. (1987). Pragmatism as a foundation for occupational therapy. *American Journal of Occupational Therapy, 41,* 522-525.

Brown, R. (1986). *Social Psychology* (2nd ed.). New York: Free Press.

Bruner, J. (1990). *Acts of Meaning.* Cambridge, MA: Harvard University Press.

Burke, J. P. (1977). A clinical perspective on motivation: Pawn versus origin. *American Journal of Occupational Therapy, 31,* 254-258.

Christiansen, C. (1981). Toward resolution of crisis: Research requisites in occupational therapy. *Occupational Therapy Journal of Research, 1,* 115-124.

Christiansen, C. (1991). Occupational therapy: Intervention for life performance. In C. Christiansen & C. Baum (Eds.), *Occupational therapy: Overcoming human performance deficits.* (pp. 1-13). Thorofare, NJ: SLACK Incorporated.

Christiansen, C. (1994). A social framework for understanding self-care intervention. In C. Christiansen (Ed.), *Ways of living: Self-care strategies for special needs.* (pp. 1-26). Rockville, MD: American Occupational Therapy Association.

Christiansen, C. (In press). Three perspectives on balance in occupation. In F. Clark & R. Zemke (Eds.), *Occupational science: The first five years.* Philadelphia: F. A. Davis.

Clark, F. A. (1993). Occupation embedded in a real life: Interweaving occupational science and occupational therapy. 1993 Eleanor Clarke Slagle Lecture. *American Journal of Occupational Therapy, 47,* 1067-1078.

Clark, F. A., Parham, D., Carlson, M. E., Frank, G., Jackson, J., Pierce, D., Wolfe, R. J., & Zemke, R. (1991). Occupational science: Academic innovation in the service of occupational therapy's future. *American Journal of Occupational Therapy, 45,* 300-310.

Cynkin, S., & Robinson, A. M. (1990). *Occupational therapy and activities health: Toward health through activities.* Boston: Little, Brown.

DiMatteo, M. R. (1991). *The psychology of health, illness, and medical care: An individual perspective.* Pacific Grove, CA: Brooks-Cole.

Dunton, W. R. (1918). The principles of occupational therapy. *Public Health Nurse, 10,* 316-321.

Englehardt, H. T. (1977). Defining occupational therapy: The meaning of therapy and the virtues of occupation. *American Journal of Occupational Therapy, 31,* 666-672.

Evans, A. K. (1987). Nationally speaking: Definition of occupation as the core concept of occupational therapy. *American Journal of Occupational Therapy, 41,* 627-628.

Fidler, G. S. (1981). From crafts to competence. *American Journal of Occupational Therapy, 35,* 567-573.

Fidler, G. S. & Fidler, J. W. (1979). Doing and becoming: purposeful action and self-actualization. *American Journal of Occupational Therapy, 32,* 305-310.

Fidler, G. S. & Fidler, J. W. (1983). Doing and becoming: The occupational therapy experience. In G. Kielhofner (Ed.), *Health through occupation.* (pp. 267-280). Philadelphia: F.A. Davis.

Frank, G. (1994). The personal meaning of self-care. In C. Christiansen (Ed.), *Ways of living: Self-care strategies for special needs.* (pp. 27-49). Rockville, MD: American Occupational Therapy Association.

Henderson, A., Cermak, S., Coster, W., Murray, E., Trombly, C., & Tickle-Degnen, L. (1991). The issue is: Occupational science is multidimensional. *American Journal of Occupational Therapy, 45,* 370-372.

Kielhofner, G. (1977). Temporal adaptation: A conceptual framework for occupational therapy. *American Journal of Occupational Therapy, 31,* 235-242.

Kielhofner, G. (1993). *Conceptual foundations of occupational therapy.* Philadelphia: F. A. Davis.

Kielhofner, G., & Burke, J. P. (1977). Occupational therapy after sixty years: An account of changing identity and knowledge. *American Journal of Occupational Therapy, 31,* 675-689.

Levine, R. (1991). Occupation as a therapeutic medium. In C. Christiansen & C. Baum (Eds.), *Occupational therapy: Overcoming human performance deficits.* (pp. 592-631). Thorofare, NJ: SLACK Incorporated.

Mattingly, C., & Fleming, M. (1993). *Clinical Reasoning.* Philadelphia: F.A. Davis.

Meyer, A. (1922). The philosophy of occupational therapy. *Archives of Occupational Therapy, 1,* 1-10.

Mosey, A. C. (1985). A monistic or pluralistic approach to professional identity. *American Journal of Occupational Therapy, 39,* 504-509.

Mosey, A. C. (1986). *Psychosocial components of occupational therapy.* New York: Raven.

Mosey, A. C. (1989). The proper focus of scientific inquiry in occupational therapy: Frames of reference. *Occupational Therapy Journal of Research, 9,* 195-201.

Mosey, A. C. (1992). Partition of occupational science and occupational therapy. *American Journal of Occupational Therapy, 46,* 851-855.

Nelson, D. L. (1988). Occupation: Form and performance. *American Journal of Occupational Therapy, 42,* 633-641.

Reilly, M. (1962). Occupation can be one of the great ideas of 20th century medicine. *American Journal of Occupational Therapy, 16,* 1-9.

Rogers, J. (1982). The spirit of independence: The evolution of a philosophy. *American Journal of Occupational Therapy, 36,* 709-715.

Rommerveit, R. (1980). On meanings of acts and what is meant and made known by what is said in a pluralistic social world. In M. Brenner (Ed.), *The structure of action.* (pp. 108-149). Oxford: Basil Blackwell.

Shannon, P .D. (1977). The derailment of occupational therapy. *American Journal of Occupational Therapy, 31,* 229-234.

Slagle, E. C. (1922). Training aids for mental patients. *Archives of Occupational Therapy, 1,* 11-17.

Tracy, S. (1910). *Studies in invalid occupations: A manual for nurses and attendants.* Boston: Whitcomb & Burrows.

Upham, E. G. (1918). *Ward occupations in hospitals. Federal Board for Vocational Education Bulletin 25.* Washington DC: Government Printing Office.

White, R. W. (1971). The urge towards competence. *American Journal of Occupational Therapy, 25,* 271-274.

Yerxa, E. (1967). Authentic occupational therapy. *American Journal of Occupational Therapy, 21,* 1-9.

Yerxa, E., Clark, F., Frank, G., Jackson, J., Parham, D., Pierce, D., Stein, C., & Zemke, R. (1989). An introduction to occupational science: A foundation for occupational therapy in the 21st century. In J. Johnson & E. Yerxa (Eds.), *Occupational science: The foundation for new models of practice.* (pp. 1-18). New York: Haworth.

❖

Prepared by Charles Christiansen, EdD, OTR, OT(C), FAOTA; Florence Clark, PhD, OTR, FAOTA; Gary Kielhofner, DPM, OTR, FAOTA; Joan Rogers, PhD, OTR, FAOTA; with contributions from David Nelson, PhD, OTR, FAOTA for the Commission on Practice (Jim Hinojosa, PhD, OTR, FAOTA, Chairperson. Adopted by the Representative Assembly 1995.

POSITION PAPER: PURPOSEFUL ACTIVITY

The American Occupational Therapy Association (AOTA) submits this paper to clarify the use of the term purposeful activity, a central focus of occupational therapy throughout its history. People engage in purposeful activity as part of their daily life routines in the context of occupational performance (AOTA, 1979). Occupation refers to active participation in self-maintenance, work, leisure, and play. Purposeful activity refers to goal-directed behaviors or tasks that comprise occupations. An activity is purposeful if the individual is an active, voluntary participant and if the activity is directed toward a goal that the individual considers meaningful (Evans, 1987; Gilfoyle, 1984; Mosey, 1986; Nelson, 1988). The purposefulness of an activity lies with the individual performing the activity and with the context in which it is done (Henderson et al., 1991). The meaning of an activity is unique to each person, influenced by his or her life experiences (Mosey, 1986; Pedretti, 1982), life roles, interests, age, and cultural background, as well as the situational context in which the activity occurs. Occupational therapy practitioners (i.e., registered occupational therapists and certified occupational therapy assistants) are committed to the use of purposeful activity to evaluate, facilitate, restore, or maintain individuals' abilities to function in their daily occupations.

Occupational therapists use activities to evaluate an individual's capacities to meet the functional demands of his or her environment and daily life. On the basis of an evaluation, the occupational therapy practitioner, in collaboration with the individual, designs activity experiences that offer the individual opportunities for effective action. Purposeful activities assist and build upon the individual's abilities and lead to achievement of personal functional goals.

Purposeful activity provides opportunities for persons to achieve mastery of their environment, and successful performance promotes feelings of personal competence (Fidler & Fidler, 1978). A person who is involved in purposeful activity directs attention to the goal rather than to the processes required for achievement of the goal. Engagement in purposeful activity within the context of interpersonal, cultural, physical, and other environmental conditions requires and elicits coordination among the individual's sensory motor, cognitive, and psychosocial systems. Purposeful activity may involve the independent use of complex cognitive processes, such as premeditation, reflection, planning, and use of symbolic cues. Conversely, it may involve less complex processes and take place in an environment of external structure, support, and supervision (Allen, 1987; Henderson et al., 1991). Engagement in purposeful activity provides direct and objective feedback of performance both to the occupational therapy practitioner and the individual.

The therapeutic purposes for which purposeful activity is used include mastery of a new skill, restoration of a deficient ability, compensation for functional disability, health maintenance, or prevention of dysfunction. To use purposeful activity therapeutically, an occupational therapy practitioner analyzes the activity from several perspectives. First, the activity is examined to identify its component parts to determine which skills and abilities are necessary to complete the task. Second, it is examined in terms of the context in which it will be performed. Third, the practitioner considers the person's age, occupational roles, cultural background, gender, interests, and preferences that may influence the meaningfulness of the activity for the individual. All this information is considered together to assist the occupational therapy practitioner in synthesizing (i.e., adapting, grading, and combining) activities for therapeutic purposes for a particular individual.

Purposeful activities cannot be prescribed on the basis of analysis of their inherent characteristics alone; rather, by definition, prescription of purposeful activity is individual-specific. An occupational therapy practitioner grades or adapts a chosen activity for an individual to promote successful performance or elicit a particular response. Grading activities challenges the patient's abilities by progressively changing the process, tools, materials, or environment of a given activity to gradually increase or decrease performance demands. These incremental modifications are made in response to the individual's dynamic changes and provide opportunities for gradual development of skill and related therapeutic benefits. The grading of activities is accomplished by modifying the sequence, duration, or procedures of the task; the individual's position; the position of the tools and materials; the size, shape, weight, or texture of the materials; the nature and degree of interpersonal contact; the extent of physical handling by the occupational therapy practitioner during performance; or the environment in which the activity is attempted. Supportive or assistive devices or techniques may be used to enhance the effectiveness of an activity or to facilitate performance (Henderson et al., 1991; Pedretti & Pasquinelli, 1990). Such techniques or devices are considered facilitative or preparatory to performance of purposeful activity and engagements in occupations.

If the therapy goal is to enhance a performance component so that an individual can engage in an occupational performance area, the selected activity and environmental conditions are manipulated to present graded challenges to the specific skills required. When an individual's successful completion of a task is a priority, occupational therapy practitioners adapt the task and the environment to facilitate performance. Adaptation is a process that changes an aspect of the activity or the environment to enable successful performance and accomplish a particular therapeutic goal. Adaptation of a task may require the use of assistive devices and techniques or grading strategies.

Occupational therapy education provides the necessary background for using activities as therapeutic modalities by instructing the student about behavioral and biological sciences related to the use and meaning of activity, about the nature of purposeful activity, and about the application of activity to therapeutic problems within occupational therapy frames of reference.

In summary, purposeful activity occurs within the context of work, self-care, play, and leisure activities and is used therapeutically to evaluate, facilitate, restore, or maintain individuals' abilities to function competently within their daily occupations. The occupational therapy practitioner's commitment to those whom he or she serves is to guide them in the use of purposeful activities so as to empower them to enhance the quality of their being in the daily reality where they live as parents, children, students, homemakers, workers, or retirees (Reilly, 1966).

References

Allen, C. K. (1987). Activity: Occupational therapy's treatment method (Slagle lecture). *American Journal of Occupational Therapy, 41,* 563-575.

American Occupational Therapy Association (1979). Resolution C, 531-79: The philosophical base of occupational therapy. *American Journal of Occupational Therapy, 33,* 785.

Evans, K. A. (1987). Nationally speaking—Definition of occupation as the core concept of occupational therapy. *American Journal of Occupational Therapy, 41,* 627-628.

Fidler, G. S., & Fidler, J. W. (1978). Doing and becoming: Purposeful action and self-actualization. *American Journal of Occupational Therapy, 38,* 305-310.

Gilfoyle, E. M. (1984). Transformation of a profession (Slagle lecture). *American Journal of Occupational Therapy, 38,* 575-584.

Henderson, A., Cermak, S., Coster, W., Murray, E., Trombly, C., & Tickle-Degnen, L. (1991). The issue is—Occupational science is multidimensional. *American Journal of Occupational Therapy, 45,* 370-372.

Mosey, A. C. (1986). *Psychosocial components of occupational therapy.* New York, NY: Raven.

Nelson, D. L. (1988). Occupation: Form and performance. *American Journal of Occupational Therapy, 42,* 633-641.

Pedretti, L. W. (1982, May). The compatibility of current treatment methods in physical disabilities with the philosophical base of occupational therapy. Paper presented at the 62nd Annual Conference of the American Occupational Therapy Association, Philadelphia, PA.

Pedretti, L. W., & Pasquinelli, S. (1990). A frame of reference for occupational therapy in physical dysfunction. In L. W. Pedretti, & B. Zoltan (Eds.), *Occupational therapy practical skills for physical dysfunction* (pp. 1-17). St. Louis, MO: Mosby.

Reilly, M. (1966). The challenge of the future to an occupational therapist. *American Journal of Occupational Therapy, 20,* 221-225.

❖

Prepared by Jim Hinojosa, PhD, OTR, FAOTA; Joyce Sabari, PhD, OTR; and Lorraine Pedretti, MS, OTR, with contributions from Mark S. Rosenfeld, PhD, OTR and Catherine Trombly, ScD, OTR/L, FAOTA, for the Commission on Practice (Jim Hinojosa, PhD, OTR, FAOTA, Chairperson).

Approved by the Representative Assembly April 1983. Revised and approved by the Representative Assembly June 1993.

Used by permission of the American Occupational Therapy Association, Inc., Rockville, MD. AOTA. (1993). Position paper on purposeful activity. *American Journal of Occupational Therapy, 47*, 1081-1082.

Position Paper: Occupational Performance: Occupational Therapy's Definition of Function

Fidler and Fidler (1963) define function as "doing"; Trombly (1993) Promotes the use of "occupational function"; and function can describe a performance (i.e., functional strength, functional range of motion, and functional skills). The word *function* can mean role, use, activity, capacity, job, position, pursuit, or place (Landau & Bogus, 1977). The many ways in which the word *function* is used, or implied, may contribute to confusion regarding occupational therapy's unique role in addressing function. Although there may be some confusion about the use of terms, there is no confusion about the sense of purpose held by occupational therapy practitioners as they address the functional needs of the clients they serve.

Occupational therapy uses the word *function* interchangeably with performance and occupational performance because occupation therapy's domain is the function of the person in his or her occupational roles. The concept of function is implicit, rather than explicit, in many of the frames of reference used by occupational therapy practitioners as they focus on strategies to overcome deficits that impair the function of the individual. Occupational therapy practitioners help people address challenges or difficulties that threaten or impair their ability to perform activities and tasks that are basic to the fulfillment of their roles as worker, parent, spouse or partner, sibling, and friend to self or others.

In order to understand how occupational therapy uses *function*, it is necessary to review the historical roots of occupat;ional therapy. Occupational therapy emerged az a developing profession in the years during and following World War I. The theoretical writings of Adolph Meyer (1922) and others were initially influenced by the then emerging school of American psychology whose "functional approach" focused on the process of adaptation to the environment rather than to the structure of the organism (Boring, 1950). The founders of occupational therapy were committed to the importance of occupation and the preservation of function (Peloquin, 1991), and early clinical efforts focused on the role of work and productivity to maintain or improve function (Hopkins, 1988). The concept of function and occupation remains at the core of occupational therapy today. However, more recently, the interaction of the functional and structural approaches has emerged, and function is viewed as the interaction of neural and physiological mechanisms, behavior, and environment. This interaction is critical to understanding the effect of occupation on health (Almli, 1993), as the function of the individual is supported in a dynamic relationship between the person, his or her occupation, and the environment (see Figure 1). The unique term used by occupational therapies to express function is *occupational performance*. "Occupational performance reflects the individual's dynamic experience of engaging in daily occupations within the environment" (Law & Baum, 1994, p. 12).

The concept of function has always been a central focus of occupational therapy and remains so. Other professions are beginning to recognize its importance and are placing increased value on function. Fisher (1992) acknowledged that the common goal of promoting functional independence is shared by occupational therapy, physical therapy, nursing, social work, psychology, and medicine, among others. A shift is occurring from a focus on pathology to a focus on function, as one of the primary indicators of treatment effectiveness (Ware, 1993). This shift also brings to the forefront the issues that occupational therapy has always valued—the person's capacity to function in a community context.

Occupational therapy's emphasis on function is broader than the function of a human organ [or body part] (Christiansen, 1991). It goes far beyond the loss or abnormality of the anatomical structure or function as defined by *impairment* (National Center for Medical Rehabilitation Research [NCMRR], 1993); or the lack of ability to perform and action or activity in the manner considered normal as defined by *functional limitation* (NCMRR). Occupational therapy views the individual as performing activities and roles within a social, cultural, and physical environment as defined by ability, or with a limitation—*disability* (NCMRR). The occupational therapy practitioner addresses the function of the individual at the occupational performance level where the environmental supports and barriers, the individual's skills, and

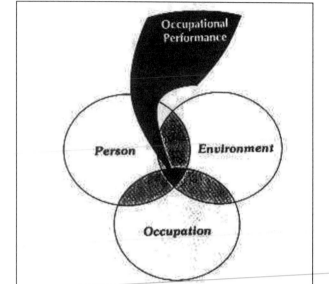

Figure 1. Reprinted with permission from Law, M. (1993). Planning for children with physical disabilities: Identifying and changing disabling environments through participatory research. Doctoral dissertation, University of Waterloo, Waterloo, Canada.

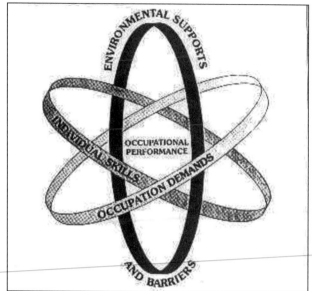

Figure 2. Reprinted with permission from Law, M., Cooper, B., Letts, L., Rigby, P., Stewart, S., & Strong, S. (1994). A model of person-environment interactions: Application to occupational therapy. Unpublished manuscript, McMaster University, Hamilton, Canada.

the individual's occupational demands interact (see Figure 2).

Since 1917, occupational therapy has focused its services to enhance the function of individuals with, or threatened with, disability. Its practitioners have focused their efforts on function by using interventions to improve the occupational performance of persons who lack the ability to perform an action or activity considered necessary for their everyday lives. This is accomplished through a joint effort of the person and the clinician, where the person's problems, strengths, and assets are identified; followed by therapeutic interventions, educational strategies, access to resources, and environmental adaptations, so the person can accomplish his or her goals (Law & Baum, 1994). The unique contribution of occupational therapy is that the practitioner creates the opportunity for individuals to gain the skill and confidence to accomplish activities and tasks that are meaningful and productive, and in doing so, increases their occupational performance, thus their function.

REFERENCES

Almli, C. R. (1993, June). *Motor system, development, and neuroplasticity: Implications of theory and practice in occupational therapy.* AOTF Research Colloquium, Seattle, WA.

Boring, E. G. (1950). *A history of experimental psychology* (2nd ed.). Englewood Cliffs, NJ: Prentice Hall.

Christiansen, C. (1991). Occupational therapy intervention for life performance. In C. Christiansen & C. M. Baum (Eds.), *Occupational therapy: Overcoming human performance deficits* (pp. 3-43). Thorofare, NJ: SLACK Incorporated.

Fidler, G., & Fidler, J. (1963). *Occupational therapy: A communication process in psychiatry.* New York: Macmillan.

Fisher, A. G. (1992). The Foundation—Functional measures, part 1: What is function, what should we measure, and how should we measure it? *American Journal of Occupational Therapy, 46,* 183 - 185.

Hopkins, H. L. (1988). An historical perspective on occupational therapy. In H. L. Hopkins & H. D.

Smith (Eds.), *Willard and Spackman's occupational therapy* (7th ed., pp. 16 - 37). Philadelphia, PA: Lippincott.

Landau, S. L., & Bogus, R. J. (1977). *The Doubleday Roget's thesaurus in dictionary form* (p. 278). Garden City, NY: Doubleday.

Law, M., & Baum, C. M. (1994). Creating the future: A Joint effort. St. Louis: Authors (Program in Occupational Therapy, Washington University School of Medicine, 4567 Scott Avenue, St. Louis, MO 63110).

Meyer, A. (1922). The philosophy of occupational therapy. *Archives of Occupational Therapy, 1* (1), 1 - 10.

National Center for Medical Rehabilitation. Research. (1993). *Research Plan for the National Center for Medical Rehabilitation Research* (National Institutes of Health Publication No. 93 - 3509). Washington, DC: U.S. Government Printing Office.

Peloquin, S. M. (1991). Looking Back—Occupational therapy service: Individual and collective understand-ing of the founders, part 1. *American Journal of Occupational Therapy, 45,* 352 - 360.

Trombly, C. (1993). The Issue Is—Anticipating the future: Assessment of occupational function. *American Journal of Occupational Therapy, 47,* 253 - 257.

Ware, J. E. (1993). Measures for a new era of health assessment. In A. L. Stewart & J. E. Ware (Eds.), *Measuring functioning and well-being* (pp. 3-12). Durham, NC: Duke University Press.

❖

Prepared by Carolyn Baum, PhD, OTR, FAOTA; Dorothy Edwards, PhD; and the faculty of the Program in Occupational Therapy, Washington University School of Medicine, St. Louis, MO, for the Commission on Practice (Jim Hinojosa, PhD, OTR, FAOTA, Chairperson).

Adopted by the Representative Assembly April 1995.

Appendix B

UNIFORM TERMINOLOGY FOR REPORTING OCCUPATIONAL THERAPY SERVICES, FIRST EDITION

INTRODUCTION

August 1978, the American Occupational Therapy Association Executive Board charged the Commission on Practice to form a Task Force to 1.) review the existing occupational therapy terminology and relative value reporting systems, and 2.) develop a proposal for a national occupational therapy product reporting system.

At the time Public Law 95-142 was passed, no national system for reporting productivity of hospital-based occupational therapy services existed. The American Occupational Therapy Association Commission on Practice OT Uniform Reporting System Task Force was created in August 1978 to develop a proposal for a national system. Sylvia Harlock, OTR (Washington), member of the AOTA Commission on Practice, was appointed by the Commission Chair John Farace, OTR, to chair the Task Force.

Members selected to serve on the Task Force were:

Mary Lou Hymen, OTR California
Kathy McFarland, OTR Washington
Kathy Saunders, OTR Wisconsin
Louise Thibodaux, OTR Alabama
Carole Hays, OTR Division on Practice, AOTA National Office

Description of Occupational Therapy Service

Given the diversity of services provided by occupational therapy, the multiplicity of evaluation and treatment procedures which may often be used to achieve the same treatment outcomes, and the lack of a uniformly used description of occupational therapy service delivery, including definitions of terminology, the Task Force first developed the Description of Occupational Therapy Services. In selecting items and defining terms, the following criteria were taken into consideration:

1. Emphasis on description of treatment outcomes rather than treatment procedures.

2. Reflection of Medicare and Medicaid guidelines in terminology and category selection and definition.

3. Comprehensive description of occupational therapy services/product.

4. Reflection of the uniqueness of occupational therapy services/product in comparison with the services of other professions.

5. Coverage of recognized occupational therapy role in medical practice rather than all possible occupational therapy roles.

OCCUPATIONAL THERAPY FUNCTION

Occupational Therapy is the application of purposeful, goal-oriented activity in the evaluation, problem identification, and/or treatment of persons whose function is impaired by physical illness or injury, emotional disorder, congenital or developmental disability, or the aging process, in order to achieve optimum functioning, to prevent disability, and to maintain health. Specific occupational therapy services include, but are not limited to, the following:

Education and training and evaluation of performance capacity in activities of daily living (ADL); the design, fabrication, and application of orthoses (splints); sensorimotor activities; guidance in selection and use of adaptive equipment; therapeutic use of activities and the activity process to develop/restore function performance; prevocational evaluation and training; consultation concerning the adaptation of physical environments for the handicapped; involvement in discharge planning and community re-entry; time/space/role management; and opportunity for self-expression and communication. These services are provided to individuals, groups, and to the community.

Occupational Therapy Services Outline

I. Occupational Therapy Assessment
  A. Screening
  B. Patient-Related Consultation
  C. Evaluation
    1. Independent Living/Daily Living Skills and Performance
    2. Sensorimotor Skill and Performance Components
    3. Cognitive Skill and Performance Components
    4. Psychosocial Skill and Performance Components
    5. Therapeutic Adaptations
    6. Specialized Evaluation
  D. Reassessment

II. Occupational Therapy Treatment
  A. Independent Living/Daily Living Skills
    1. Physical Daily Living Skills
      a. Grooming and Hygiene
      b. Feeding/Eating
      c. Dressing
      d. Functional Mobility
      e. Functional Communication
      f. Object Manipulation
    2. Psychological/Emotional Daily Living Skills
      a. Self-Concept/Self-Identity
      b. Situational Coping
      c. Community Involvement
    3. Work
      a. Homemaking
      b. Child Care/Parenting
      c. Employment Preparation
    4. Play/Leisure
  B. Sensorimotor Components
    1. Neuromuscular
      a. Reflex Integration
      b. Range of Motion
      c. Gross and Fine Coordination
      d. Strength and Endurance
    2. Sensory Integration
      a. Sensory Awareness
      b. Visual-Spatial Awareness
      c. Body Integration
  C. Cognitive Components
    1. Orientation
    2. Conceptualization/Comprehension
      a. Concentration
      b. Attention Span
      c. Memory
    3. Cognitive Integration
      a. Generalization
      b. Problem Solving
  D. Psychosocial Components
    1. Self-Management
      a. Self-Expression
      b. Self-Control
    2. Dyadic Interaction
    3. Group Interaction
  E. Therapeutic Adaptation
    1. Orthotics
    2. Prosthetics
    3. Assistive/Adaptive Equipment

F. Prevention
1. Energy Conservation
2. Joint Protection/Body Mechanics
3. Positioning
4. Coordination of Daily Living Activities

III. Patient/Client-Related Conferences
A. Professional Conferences
B. Agency Conferences
C. Patient/Client-Advocate Conferences

IV. Travel: Patient-Treatment Related

The following items do not involve direct patient care.
V. Service Management
A. Quality Review/Maintenance of Quality
1. Development of Standards of Quality Treatment/Services
2. Chart Audit
3. Accrediting Reviews
4. Occupational Therapy Care Review
5. Inservice Education
B. Departmental Maintenance
C. Employee Meetings
D. Program-Related Conferences
E. Supervision

VI. Education
A. Occupational Therapy Clinical Education: Occupational Therapy Students
B. Occupational Therapy Clinical Education: Others
C. Continuing Education

VII. Research

OCCUPATIONAL THERAPY SERVICES DESCRIPTION

I. Occupational Therapy Assessment
Occupational therapy assessment refers to the process of determining the need for, nature of, and estimated time of treatment, determining the needed coordination with other persons involved, and documenting these activities.

A. *Screening*

Screening refers to the review of potential patient's/client's case to determine the need for evaluation and treatment. It includes discussion with other professionals and/or patient advocate, and patient/client interview or administration of screening tool.

B. *Patient-Related Consultation*

Patient-related consultation refers to the sharing of relevant information with other professionals of patients/clients who are not currently referred to occupational therapy. This may include but is not limited to discussion, chart review, treatment recommendation, and documentation.

C. *Evaluation*

Evaluation refers to the process of obtaining and interpreting data necessary for treatment. This includes planning for and documenting the evaluation process and results. This data may be gathered through record review, specific observation, interview, and the administration of data collection procedures. Such procedures include but are not limited to the use of standardized tests, performance checklists, and activities and tasks designed to evaluate specific performance abilities. Categories of occupational therapy evaluation include the independent living/daily living skills and performance and their components.

1. *Independent Living/Daily Living Skills and Performance (see IIA).*
2. *Sensorimotor Skill and Performance Components (see IIB).*
3. *Cognitive Skill and Performance Components (see IIC).*
4. *Psychosocial Skill and Performance Components (see IID).*
5. *Therapeutic Adaptations (see IIE).*
6. *Specialized Evaluations*

Specialized evaluations refer to evaluations or tests requiring specialized training and/or advanced education to administer and interpret. Examples of specialized evaluations are employment preparation, evaluation (prevocational testing), sensory integration evaluation, prosthetic evaluation, driver's training evaluation.

D. *Reassessment*

Reassessment refers to the process of obtaining and interpreting data necessary for updating treatment plans and goals. This frequently involves administering only portions of the initial evaluation, documenting results, and/or revising treatment.

II. *Occupational Therapy Treatment*

Occupational therapy treatment refers to the use of specific activities or methods to develop, improve, and/or restore the performance of necessary functions; compensate for dysfunction and/or minimize debilitation; and the planning for and documenting of treatment performance. The necessary functions treated in occupational therapy are the following:

A. *Independent Living/Daily Living Skills*

1. *Physical Daily Living Skills*

Physical daily living skills refer to the skill and performance of daily personal care, with or without adaptive equipment. It includes but is not limited to:

a. *Grooming and Hygiene*
Grooming and hygiene refer to the skill and performance of personal health needs, such as bathing, toileting, hair care, shaving, applying make-up.

b. *Feeding/Eating*
Feeding/eating refers to the skill and performance of sequentially feeding oneself, including sucking, chewing, swallowing, and using appropriate utensils.

c. *Dressing*
Dressing refers to the skill and performance of choosing appropriate clothing, dressing oneself in a sequential fashion, including fastening and adjusting clothing.

d. *Functional Mobility*
Functional mobility refers to the skill and performance in moving oneself from one position or place to another. It includes skills necessary for activities such as bed mobility, wheelchair mobility, transfers (bed, car, tub, toilet, chair), and functional ambulation, with or without adaptive aids. It also includes use of public and private travel systems, such as driving own automobile and using public transportation.

e. *Functional Communication*
Functional communication refers to the skill and performance in using equipment or systems to enhance or provide communication, such as writing equipment, typewriters, letterboards, telephone, Braille writers, artificial vocalization systems, and computers.

f. *Object Manipulation*
Object manipulation refers to the skill and performance in handling large and small common objects, such as calculators, keys, money, light switches, doorknobs, and packages.

2. *Psychological/Emotional Daily Living Skills*

Psychological/emotional daily living skills refers to the skill and performance in developing one's self-concept/self-identity, coping with life situations, and participating in one's organizational and community environment. It includes but is not limited to:

a. *Self-Concept/Self-Identity*
Self-concept/self-identity refers to the cognitive image of one's functional self. This includes but is not limited to:
(1) Clearly perceiving one's needs, feelings, conflicts, values, beliefs, expectations, sexuality, and power.
(2) Realistically perceiving one's needs, feelings, conflicts, values, beliefs, expectations, sexuality, and power.
(3) Knowing one's performance strengths and limitations.
(4) Sensing one's competence, achievement, self-esteem, and self-respect.
(5) Integrating new experiences with established self-concept/self-identity.
(6) Having a sense of psychological safety and security.
(7) Perceiving one's goals and directions.

b. *Situational Coping*

Situational coping refers to skill and performance in handling stress and dealing with problems and changes in a manner that is functional for self and others. This includes but is not limited to:

(1) Setting goals, selecting, harmonizing, and managing activities of daily living to promote optimal performance.

(2) Testing goals and perceptions against reality.

(3) Perceiving changes and need for changes in self and environment.

(4) Directing and redirecting energy to overcome problems.

(5) Initiating, implementing, and following through on decisions.

(6) Assuming responsibility for self and consequences of actions.

(7) Interacting with others, dyadic and group.

c. *Community Involvement*

Community involvement refers to skill and performance in interacting within one's social system. This includes but is not limited to:

(1) Understanding social norms and their impact on society.

(2) Planning, organizing, and executing daily life activities in relationship to society, including such activities as budgeting, time management, social role management, arranging for housing, nutritional planning, assessing and using community resources.

(3) Recognizing and responding to needs to families, groups, and complex social units.

(4) Understanding and responding to organizational/community role expectations as both recipient and contributor.

3. *Work*

Work refers to skill and performance in participating in socially purposeful and productive activities. These activities may take place in the home, employment setting, school, or community. They include but are not limited to:

a. *Homemaking*

Homemaking refers to skill and performance in homemaking and home management tasks, such as meal planning, meal preparation and clean-up, laundry, cleaning, minor household repairs, shopping, and use of household safety principles.

b. *Child Care/Parenting*

Child care/parenting refers to skill and performance in child care activities and management. This includes but is not limited to physical care of children, and use of age-appropriate activities, communication, and behavior to facilitate child development.

c. *Employment Preparation*

Employment preparation refers to skill and performance in precursory job activities (including prevocational activities). This includes but is not limited to:

(1) Job acquisition skills and performance.

(2) Organizational and team participatory skills and performance.

(3) Work process skills and performance.

(4) Work product quality.

4. *Play/Leisure*

Play/leisure refers to skill and performance in choosing, performing, and engaging in activities for amusement, relaxation, spontaneous enjoyment, and/or self-expression. This includes but is not limited to:

a. Recognizing one's specific needs, interests, and adaptations necessary for performance.

b. Identifying characteristics of activities and social situations that make them play for the individual.

c. Identifying activities that contain those characteristics.

d. Choosing play activities for participation, such as sports, games, hobbies, music, drama, and other activities.

e. Testing out and adapting activities to enable participation.

f. Identifying and using community resources.

B. *Sensorimotor Components*

Sensorimotor components refer to the skill and performance of patterns of sensory and motor behavior that are prerequisites to self-care, work, and play/leisure performance. The components in this section include neuromuscular and sensory integrative skills, including perceptual motor skills.

1. *Neuromuscular*

Neuromuscular refers to the skill and performance of motor aspects of behavior. This includes but is not limited to:

a. *Reflex Integration*

Reflex integration refers to skill and performance in enhancing and supporting functional neuromuscular development through eliciting and/or inhibiting stereotyped, patterned, and/or involuntary responses coordinated at subcortical and cortical levels.

b. *Range of Motion*

Range of motion refers to skill and performance in using maximum span of joint movement in activities with and without assistance to enhance functional performance. The standard levels of performance include:

(1) Active range of motion: movement by patient, unassisted through a complete range of motion.

(2) Passive range of motion: movement performed by someone other than patient or by a mechanical device, requiring no muscle contraction on the part of the patient.

(3) Active-assistive range of motion: movement performed by the patient to the limit of his/her ability, and then completed with assistance.

c. *Gross and Fine Coordination*

Gross and fine coordination refers to skill and performance in muscle control, coordination, and dexterity while participating in activities.

(1) Muscle control: refers to skill and performance in directing muscle movement.

(2) Coordination: refers to skill and performance in gross motor activities using several muscle groups.

(3) Dexterity: refers to skill and performance in tasks using small muscle groups.

d. *Strength and Endurance*

Strength and endurance refers to skill and performance in using muscular force within time periods necessary for purposeful task performance. This involves but is not limited to progressively building strength and cardia and pulmonary reserve, increasing the length of work periods, and decreasing fatigue and strain.

2. *Sensory Integration*

Sensory integration refers to skill and performance in development and coordination of sensory input, motor output, and sensory feedback. This includes but is not limited to:

a. *Sensory Awareness*

Sensory awareness refers to skill and performance in perceiving and differentiating external and internal stimuli, such as:

(1) Tactile awareness: the perception and interpretation of stimuli through skin contact.

(2) Stereognosis: the identification of forms and nature of objects through the sense of touch.

(3) Kinesthesia: the conscious perception of muscular motion, weight, and position.

(4) Proprioceptive awareness: the identification of the positions of body parts in space.

(5) Ocular control: the localization and visual tracking of stimuli.

(6) Vestibular awareness: the detention of motion and gravitational pull as related to one's performance in functional activities, ambulation, and balance.

(7) Auditory awareness: the differentiation and identification of sounds.

(8) Gustatory awareness: the differentiation and identification of tastes.

(9) Olfactory awareness: the differentiation and identification of smells.

b. *Visual-Spatial Awareness*

Visual-spatial awareness refers to skill and performance in perceiving distances between and relationships among objects, including self. This includes but is not limited to:

(1) Figure-ground: recognition of forms and objects when presented in a configuration with competing stimuli.

(2) Form constancy: recognition of forms and objects as the same when presented in different contexts.

(3) Position in space: knowledge of one's position in space relative to other objects.

c. *Body Integration*

Body integration refers to skill and performance in perceiving and regulating the position of various muscles and body parts in relationship to each other during static and movement states. This includes but is not limited to:

(1) Body schema: refers to the perception of one's physical self through proprioceptive and interoceptive sensations.

(2) Postural balance: refers to skill and performance in developing and maintaining body posture while sitting, standing, or engaging in activity.

(3) Bilateral motor coordination: refers to skill and performance in purpose.

(4) Right-left discrimination: refers to skill and performance in differentiating right from left and vice versa.

(5) Visual-motor integration: refers to skill and performance in combining visual input with purposeful voluntary movement of the hand and other body parts involved in an activity. Visual-motor integration includes eye-hand coordination.

(6) Crossing the midline: refers to skill and performance in crossing the vertical midline of the body.

(7) Praxis: refers to skill and performance of purposeful movement that involves motor planning.

C. *Cognitive Components*

Cognitive components refer to skill and performance of the mental processes necessary to know or apprehend by understanding. This includes but is not limited to:

1. *Orientation*

Orientation refers to skill and performance in comprehending, defining, and adjusting oneself in an environment with regard to time, place, and person.

2. *Conceptualization/Comprehension*

Conceptualization/comprehension refers to skill and performance in conceiving and understanding concepts or tasks such as color identification, word recognition, sign concepts, sequencing, matching, association, classification, and abstracting. This includes but is not limited to:

a. *Concentration*

Concentration refers to skill and performance in focusing on a designated task or concept.

b. *Attention Span*

Attention span refers to skill and performance in focusing on a task or concept for a particular length of time.

c. *Memory*

Memory refers to skill and performance in retaining and recalling tasks or concepts from the past.

3. *Cognitive Integration*

Cognitive integration refers to skill and performance in applying diverse knowledge to environmental situations. This involves but is not limited to:

a. *Generalization*

Generalization refers to skill and performance in applying specific concepts to a variety of related situations.

b. *Problem Solving*

Problem solving refers to skill and performance in identifying and organizing solutions to difficulties. It includes but is not limited to:

(1) Defining or evaluating the problem.

(2) Organizing a plan.

(3) Making decisions/judgments.

(4) Implementing plan, including following through in logical sequence.

(5) Evaluating decision/judgment and plan.

D. *Psychosocial Components*

Psychosocial components refer to skill and performance in self-management, dyadic and group interaction.

1. *Self-Management*

Self-management refers to skill and performance in expressing and controlling oneself in functional and creative activities.

a. *Self-Expression*

Self-expression refers to skill and performance in perceiving one's feelings and interpreting and using a variety of communication signs and symbols. This includes but is not limited to:

(1) Experiencing and recognizing a range of emotions.

(2) Having an adequate vocabulary.

(3) Having writing and speaking skills.

(4) Interpreting and using correctly an adequate range of nonverbal signs and symbols.

b. *Self-Control*

Self-control refers to skill and performance in modulating and modifying present behaviors, and in initiating new behaviors in accordance with situational demands. It includes but is not limited to:

(1) Observing own and other's behavior.

(2) Conceptualizing problems in terms of needed behavioral changes or action.

(3) Imitating new behaviors.

(4) Directing and redirecting energies into stress-reducing activities and behaviors.

2. *Dyadic Interaction*

Dyadic interaction refers to skill and performance in relating to another person. This includes but is not limited to:

a. Understanding social/cultural norms of communication and interaction in various activity
and social situations.

b. Setting limits on self and others.

c. Compromising and negotiating.

d. Handling competition, frustration, anxiety, success, and failure.

e. Cooperating and competing with others.

f. Responsibly relying on self and others.

3. *Group Interaction*

Group interaction refers to skill and performance in relating to groups of three to six persons, or larger. This includes but is not limited to:

a. Knowing and performing a variety of task and social/emotional role behaviors.

b. Understanding common stages of group process.

c. Participating in a group in a manner that is mutually beneficial to self and others.

E. *Therapeutic Adaptation*

Therapeutic adaptations refer to the design and/or restructuring of the physical environment to assist self-care, work, and play/leisure performance. This includes selecting, obtaining, fitting and fabricating equipment, and instructing the client, family and/or staff in proper use and care of equipment. It also includes minor repair and modification for correct fit, position, or use. Categories of therapeutic adaptations consist of:

1. *Orthotics*

Orthotics refer to the provision of dynamic and static splints, braces, and slings for the purpose of relieving pain, maintaining joint alignment, protecting joint integrity, improving function, and/or decreasing deformity.

2. *Prosthetics*

Prosthetics refer to the training in use of artificial substitutes of missing body parts, which augment performance of function.

3. *Assistive/Adaptive Equipment*

Assistive/adaptive equipment refers to the provision of special devices that assist in performance and/or structural or positional changes such as the installation of ramps, bars, changes in furniture heights, adjustments of traffic patterns, and modifications of wheelchairs.

F. *Prevention*

Prevention refers to skill and performance in minimizing debilitation. It may include programs for persons where predisposition to disability exists, as well as for those who have already incurred a disability. This includes but is not limited to:

1. *Energy Conservation*

Energy conservation refers to skill and performance in applying energy-saving procedures, activity restriction, work simplification, time management, and/or organization of the environment to minimize energy output.

2. *Joint Protection/Body Mechanics*

Joint protection/body mechanics refers to skill and performance in applying principles or procedures to minimize stress on joints. Procedures may include the use of proper body mechanics, avoidance of static or deforming postures, and/or avoidance of excessive weight-bearing.

3. *Positioning*

Positioning refers to skill and performance in the placement of a body part in alignment to promote optimal functioning.

4. *Coordination of Daily Living Activities*

Coordination of daily living activities refers to skill and performance in selecting and coordinating activities of self-care, work, play/leisure, and rest to promote optimal performance of daily life tasks.

III. *Patient/Client-Related Conferences*

Patient/client-related conferences include participating in meetings to discuss and identify needs, treatment program, and future plans of referred client and documenting such participation. Patient/client may or may not be present. Categories of conferences include:

A. *Professional Conferences*

Professional conferences refer to participating in meetings with a group or individual professionals to discuss patient's/client's status, and to advise/consult regarding treatment needs. Synonymous terms for professional conferences include initial conference, interim review, discharge planning, case conference, and others.

B. *Agency Conferences*

Agency conferences refer to participating in meetings with vocational, social, religious, recreational health, educational, and other community representatives to assess, implement, or coordinate the use of services.

C. *Patient/Client-Advocate Conferences*

Patient/client-advocate conferences refer to participating in meetings with client advocate (e.g., family, guardian, or others responsible for patient/client) to assess patient's/client's situation, set goals, plan treatment and/or discharge; and/or to instruct client advocate to support or carry out treatment program.

IV. *Travel: Patient-Treatment Related*

Travel: patient-treatment related refers to travel by therapists, with or without patient; that is, related to direct patient treatment.

❖

Commission on Practice, the American Occupational Therapy Association, Inc.

Adopted March 1979 by the Representative Assembly, AOTA.

Used by permission of the American Occupational Therapy Association, Inc., Rockville, MD.

UNIFORM TERMINOLOGY FOR OCCUPATIONAL THERAPY, THIRD EDITION

This is an official document of the American Occupational Therapy Association. This document is intended to provide a generic outline of the domain of concern of occupational therapy and is designed to create common terminology for the profession and to capture the essence of occupational therapy succinctly for others.

It is recognized that the phenomena that constitute the profession's domain of concern can be categorized, and labeled, in a number of different ways. This document is not meant to limit those in the field, formulating theories or frames of reference, who may wish to combine or refine particular constructs. It is also not meant to limit those who would like to conceptualize the profession's domain of concern in a different manner.

INTRODUCTION

The first edition of Uniform Terminology was approved and published in 1979 (AOTA, 1979). In 1989, the Uniform Terminology for Occupational Therapy, Second Edition (AOTA, 1989) was approved and published. The second document presented an organized structure for understanding the areas of practice for the profession of occupational therapy. The document outlined two domains. Performance Areas (activities of daily living [ADL], work and productive activities, and play or leisure) include activities that the occupational therapy practitioner1 emphasizes when determining functional abilities. Performance Components (sensorimotor, cognitive, psychosocial, and psychological

aspects) are the elements of performance that occupational therapists assess and, when needed, in which they intervene for improved performance.

This third edition has been further expanded to reflect current practice and to incorporate contextual aspects of performance. Performance Areas, Performance Components, and Performance Contexts are the parameters of occupational therapy's domain of concern. Performance areas are broad categories of human activity that are typically part of daily life. They are activities of daily living, work and productive activities, and play or leisure activities. Performance components are fundamental human abilities that-to varying degrees and in differing combinations-are required for successful engagement in performance areas. These components are sensorimotor, cognitive, and psychosocial and psychological. Performance contexts are situations or factors that influence an individual's engagement in desired and/or required performance areas. Performance contexts consist of temporal aspects (chronological, developmental, life cycle, and disability status) and environmental aspects (physical, social, and cultural). There is an interactive relationship among performance areas, performance components, and performance contexts. Function in performance areas is the ultimate concern of occupational therapy, with performance components considered as they relate to participation in performance areas. Performance areas and performance components are always viewed within performance contexts. Performance contexts are taken into consideration when determining function and dysfunction relative to performance areas and performance components, and in planning intervention. For example, the occupational therapist does not evaluate strength (a performance component) in isolation. Strength is considered as it affects necessary or desired tasks (performance areas). If the individual is interested in homemaking, the occupational therapy practitioner would consider the interaction of strength with homemaking tasks. Strengthening could be addressed through kitchen activities, such as cooking and putting groceries away. In some cases, the practitioner would employ an adaptive approach and recommend that the family switch from heavy stoneware to lighter weight dishes, or use lighter weight pots on the stove to enable the individual to make dinner safely without becoming fatigued or compromising safety.

Occupational therapy assessment involves examining performance areas, performance components, and performance contexts. Intervention may be directed toward elements of performance areas (e.g., dressing, vocational exploration), performance components (e.g., endurance, problem solving), or the environmental aspects of performance contexts. In the last case, the physical and/or social environment may be altered or augmented to improve and/or maintain function. After identifying the performance areas the individual wishes or needs to address, the occupational therapist assesses the features of the environments in which the tasks will be performed. If an individual's job requires cooking in a restaurant as opposed to leisure cooking at home, the occupational therapy practitioner faces several challenges to enable the individual's success in different environments. Therefore, the third critical aspect of performance is the performance context, the features of the environment that affect the person's ability to engage in functional activities.

This document categorizes specific activities in each of the performance areas (ADL, work and productive activities, play or leisure). This categorization is based on what is considered "typical", and is not meant to imply that a particular individual characterizes personal activities in the same manner as someone else. Occupational therapy practitioners embrace individual differences, and so would document the unique pattern of the individual being served, rather than forcing the "typical" pattern on

him or her and family. For example, because of experience or culture, a particular individual might think of home management as an ADL task rather than "work and productive activities" (current listing). Socialization might be considered part of play or leisure activity instead of its current listing as part of "activities of daily living", because of life experience or cultural heritage.

EXAMPLES OF USE IN PRACTICE

Uniform Terminology, Third Edition defines occupational therapy's domain of concern, which includes performance areas, performance components, and performance contexts. While this document may be used by occupational therapy practitioners in a number of different areas (e.g., practice, documentation, charge systems, education, program development, marketing, research, disability classifications, and regulations), it focuses on the use of Uniform Terminology in practice. This document is not intended to define specific occupational therapy interventions. Examples of how performance areas, performance components, and performance contexts translate into practice are provided below.

❖ An individual who is injured on the job may have the potential to return to work and productive activities, which is a performance area. In order to achieve the outcome of returning to work and productive activities, the individual may need to address specific performance components such as strength, endurance, soft tissue integrity, time management, and the physical features of performance contexts, like structures and objects in his or her environment. The occupational therapy practitioner, in collaboration with the individual and other members of the vocational team, uses planned interventions to achieve the desired outcome. These interventions may include activities such as an exercise program, body mechanics instruction, and job site modifications, all of which may be provided in a work-hardening program.

❖ An elderly individual recovering from a cerebral vascular accident may wish to live in a community setting, which combines the performance areas of ADL with work and productive activities. In order to achieve the outcome of community living, the individual may need to address specific performance components, such as muscle tone, gross motor coordination, postural control, and self-management. It is also necessary to consider the sociocultural and physical features of performance contexts, such as support available from other persons, and adaptations of structures and objects within the environment. The occupational therapy practitioner, in cooperation with the team, utilizes planned interventions to achieve the desired outcome. Interventions may include neuromuscular facilitation, practice of object manipulation, and instruction in the use of adaptive equipment and home safety equipment. The practitioner and individual also pursue the selection and training of a personal assistant to ensure the completion of ADL tasks. These interventions may be provided in a comprehensive inpatient rehabilitation unit.

❖ A child with learning disabilities is required to perform educational activities within a public school setting. Engaging in educational activities is considered the performance area of work and productive activities for this child. To achieve the educational outcome of efficient and effective completion of written classroom work, the child may need to address specific performance components. These include sensory processing, perceptual skills, postural control, motor skills, and the physical features of performance contexts, such as objects (e.g., desk, chair) in the environment. In cooperation with the team, occupational therapy interventions may include activities like adapting the student's seating in the classroom to improve postural control and stability, and practicing motor control and coordination. This program could be developed by an occupational therapist and supported by school district personnel.

❖ The parents of an infant with cerebral palsy may ask to facilitate the child's involvement in the performance areas of activities of daily living and play. Subsequent to assessment, the therapist identifies specific performance components, such as sensory awareness and neuromuscular control. The practitioner also addresses the physical and cultural features of performance contexts. In collaboration with the parents, occupational therapy interventions may include activities such as seating and positioning for play, neuromuscular facilitation techniques to enable eating, facilitating parent skills in caring for and playing with their infant, and modifying the play space for accessibility. These interventions may be provided in a home-based occupational therapy program.

❖ An adult with schizophrenia may need and want to live independently in the community, which represents the performance areas of activities of daily living, work and productive activities, and leisure activities. The specific performance categories may be medication routine, functional mobility, home management, vocational exploration, play or leisure performance, and social interaction. In order to achieve the outcome of living independently, the individual may need to address specific performance components such as topographical orientation, memory, categorization, problem solving, interests, social conduct, time management, and sociocultural features of performance contexts, such as social factors (e.g., influence of family and friends) and roles. The occupational therapy practitioner, in cooperation with the team, utilizes planned interventions to achieve the desired outcome. Interventions may include activities such as training in the use of public transportation, instruction in budgeting skills, selection of and participation in social activities, and instruction in social conduct. These interventions may be provided in a community-based mental health program.

❖ An individual with a history of substance abuse may need to reestablish family roles and responsibilities, which represent the performance areas of activities of daily living, work and productive activities, and leisure activities. In order to achieve the outcome of family

I. Performance Areas

A. Activities of Daily Living
  1. Grooming
  2. Oral Hygiene
  3. Bathing/Showering
  4. Toilet Hygiene
  5. Personal Device Care
  6. Dressing
  7. Feeding and Eating
  8. Medication Routine
  9. Health Maintenance
  10. Socialization
  11. Functional Communication
  12. Functional Mobility
  13. Community Mobility
  14. Emergency Response
  15. Sexual Expression

B. Work and Productive Activities
  1. Home Management
    a. Clothing Care
    b. Cleaning
    c. Meal Preparation/Cleanup
    d. Shopping
    e. Money Management
    f. Household Maintenance
    g. Safety Procedures
  2. Care of Others
  3. Educational Activities
  4. Vocational Activities
    a. Vocational Exploration
    b. Job Acquisition
    c. Work or Job Performance
    d. Retirement Planning
    e. Volunteer Participation

C. Play or Leisure Activities
  1. Play or Leisure Exploration
  2. Play or Leisure Performance

II. Performance Components

A. Sensorimotor Components
  1. Sensory
    a. Sensory Awareness
    b. Sensory Processing
      (1) Tactile
      (2) Proprioceptive
      (3) Vestibular
      (4) Visual
      (5) Auditory
      (6) Gustatory
      (7) Olfactory
    c. Perceptual Processing
      (1) Stereognosis
      (2) Kinesthesia
      (3) Pain Response
      (4) Body Scheme
      (5) Right-Left Discrimination
      (6) Form Constancy
      (7) Position in Space
      (8) Visual-Closure
      (9) Figure Ground
      (10) Depth Perception
      (11) Spatial Relations
      (12) Topographical Orientation
  2. Neuromusculoskeletal
    a. Reflex
    b. Range of Motion
    c. Muscle Tone
    d. Strength
    e. Endurance
    f. Postural Control
    g. Postural Alignment
    h. Soft Tissue Integrity
  3. Motor
    a. Gross Coordination
    b. Crossing the Midline
    c. Laterality
    d. Bilateral Integration
    e. Motor Control
    f. Praxis
    g. Fine Motor Coordination/ Dexterity
    h. Visual-Motor Integration
    i. Oral-Motor Control

B. Cognitive Integration and Cognitive Components
  1. Level of Arousal
  2. Orientation
  3. Recognition
  4. Attention Span
  5. Initiation of Activity
  6. Termination of Activity
  7. Memory
  8. Sequencing
  9. Categorization
  10. Concept Formation
  11. Spatial Operations
  12. Problem Solving
  13. Learning
  14. Generalization

C. Psychosocial Skills and Psychological Components
  1. Psychological
    a. Values
    b. Interests
    c. Self-Concept
  2. Social
    a. Role Performance
    b. Social Conduct
    c. Interpersonal Skills
    d. Self-Expression
  3. Self-Management
    a. Coping Skills
    b. Time Management
    c. Self-Control

III. Performance Contexts

A. Temporal Aspects
  1. Chronological
  2. Developmental
  3. Life Cycle
  4. Disability Status

B. Environmental Aspects
  1. Physical
  2. Social
  3. Cultural

participation, the individual may need to address the performance components of roles, values, social conduct, self-expression, coping skills, self-control, and the sociocultural features of performance contexts, such as custom, behavior, rules, and rituals. The occupational therapy practitioner, in cooperation with the team, utilizes planned intervention to achieve the desired outcomes. Interventions may include roles and values exercises, instruction in stress management techniques, identification of family roles and activities, and support to develop family leisure routines. These interventions may be provided in an inpatient acute care unit.

PERSON-ACTIVITY-ENVIRONMENT FIT

Person-activity-environment fit refers to the match among skills and abilities of the individual; the demands of the activity; and the characteristics of the physical, social, and cultural environments. It is the interaction among the performance areas, performance components, and performance contexts that is important and determines the success of the performance. When occupational therapy practitioners provide services, they attend to all of these aspects of performance and the interaction among them. They also attend to each individual's unique personal history. The personal history includes one's skills and abilities (performance components), the past performance of specific life tasks (performance areas), and experience within particular environments (performance contexts). In addition to personal history, anticipated life tasks and role demands influence performance.

When considering the person-activity-environment fit, variables such as novelty, importance, motivation, activity tolerance, and quality are salient. Situations range from those that are completely familiar, to those that are novel and have never been experienced. Both the novelty and familiarity within a situation contribute to the overall task performance. In each situation, there is an optimal level of novelty that engages the individual sufficiently and provides enough information to perform the task. When too little novelty is present, the individual may miss cues and opportunities to perform. When too much novelty is present, the individual may become confused and distracted, inhibiting effective task performance.

Humans determine that some stimuli and situations are more meaningful than others. Individuals perform tasks they deem important. It is critical to identify what the individual wants or needs to do when planning interventions.

The level of motivation an individual demonstrates to perform a particular task is determined by both internal and external factors. An individual's biobehavioral state (e.g., amount of rest, arousal, tension) contributes to the potential to be responsive. The features of the social and physical environments (e.g., persons in the room, noise level) provide information that is either adequate or inadequate to produce a motivated state.

Activity tolerance is the individual's ability to sustain a purposeful activity over time. Individuals must not only select, initiate, and terminate activities, but they must also attend to a task for the needed length of time to complete the task and accomplish their goals.

The quality of performance is measured by standards generated by both the individual and others in the social and cultural environments in which the performance occurs. Quality is a continuum of expectations set within particular activities and contexts.

UNIFORM TERMINOLOGY FOR OCCUPATIONAL THERAPY, THIRD EDITION

"Occupational Therapy" is the use of purposeful activity or interventions to promote health and achieve functional outcomes. "Achieving functional outcomes" means to develop, improve, or restore the highest possible level of independence of any individual who is limited by a physical injury or illness, a dysfunctional condition, a cognitive impairment, a psychosocial dysfunction, a mental illness, a developmental or learning disability, or an adverse environmental condition. Assessment means the use of skilled observation or evaluation by the administration and interpretation of standardized or nonstandardized tests and measurements to identify areas for occupational therapy services.

Occupational therapy services include, but are not limited to:

1. The assessment, treatment, and education of or consultation with the individual, family, or other persons

2. Interventions directed toward developing, improving, or restoring daily living skills; work readiness or work performance; play skills or leisure capacities; or enhancing educational performances skills

3. Providing for the development, improvement, or restoration of sensorimotor, oral-motor, perceptual or neuromuscular functioning; or emotional, motivational, cognitive, or psychosocial components of performance.

These services may require assessment of the need for and use of interventions such as the design, development, adaptation, application, or training in the use of assistive technology devices; the design, fabrication, or application of rehabilitative technology such as selected orthotic devices; training in the use of assistive technology, orthotic or prosthetic devices; the application of physical agent modalities as an adjunct to or in preparation for purposeful activity; the use of ergonomic principles; the adaptation of environments and processes to enhance functional performance; or the promotion of health and wellness (AOTA, 1993, p. 1117).

I. Performance Areas

Throughout this document, activities have been described as if individuals performed the tasks themselves. Occupational therapy also recognizes that individuals arrange for tasks to be done through others. The profession views independence as the ability to self-determine activity performance, regardless of who actually performs the activity.

A. *Activities of Daily Living*—Self-maintenance tasks.
 1. *Grooming*—Obtaining and using supplies; removing body hair (use of razors, tweezers, lotions, etc.); applying and removing cosmetics; washing, drying, combing, styling, and brushing hair; caring for nails (hands and feet); caring for skin, ears, and eyes; and applying deodorant.

2. *Oral Hygiene*—Obtaining and using supplies; cleaning mouth; brushing and flossing teeth; or removing, cleaning, and reinserting dental orthotics and prosthetics.

3. *Bathing/Showering*—Obtaining and using supplies; soaping, rinsing, and drying all body parts; maintaining bathing position; transferring to and from bathing positions.

4. *Toilet Hygiene*—Obtaining and using supplies; clothing management; maintaining toileting position; transferring to and from toileting position; cleaning body; and caring for menstrual and continence needs (including catheters, colostomies, and suppository management).

5. *Personal Device Care*—Cleaning and maintaining personal care items, such as hearing aids, contact lenses, glasses, orthotics, prosthetics, adaptive equipment, and contraceptive and sexual devices.

6. *Dressing*—Selecting clothing and accessories appropriate for the time of day, weather, and occasion; obtaining clothing from storage area; dressing and undressing in a sequential fashion; fastening and adjusting clothing and shoes; and applying and removing personal devices, prostheses, or orthoses.

7. *Feeding and Eating*—Setting up food; selecting and using appropriate utensils and tableware; bringing food or drink to mouth; sucking, masticating, coughing, and swallowing; and management of alternative methods of nourishment.

8. *Medication Routine*—Obtaining medication, opening and closing containers, following prescribed schedules, taking correct quantities, reporting problems and adverse effects, and administering correct quantities using prescribed methods.

9. *Health Maintenance*—Developing and maintaining routines for illness prevention and wellness promotion, such as physical fitness, nutrition, and decreasing health risk behaviors.

10. *Socialization*—Accessing opportunities and interacting with other people in appropriate contextual and cultural ways to meet emotional and physical needs.

11. *Functional Communication*—Using equipment or systems to send and receive information, such as writing equipment, telephones, typewriters, communication boards, call lights, emergency systems, Braille writers, telecommunication devices for the deaf, and augmentative communication systems.

12. *Functional Mobility*—Moving from one position or place to another, such as in-bed mobility, wheelchair mobility, transfers (wheelchair, bed, car, tub/shower, toilet, chair, floor); performing functional ambulation and transporting objects.

13. *Community Mobility*—Moving self in the community and using public or private transportation, such as driving, or accessing buses, taxi cabs, or other public transportation systems.

14. *Emergency Response*—Recognizing sudden, unexpected hazardous situations, and initiating action to reduce the threat to health and safety.

15. *Sexual Expression*—Engaging in desired sexual activities.

B. *Work and Productive Activities*—Purposeful activities for self-development, social contribution, and livelihood.

1. *Home Management*—Obtaining and maintaining personal and household possessions and environment.

    a. *Clothing Care*—Obtaining and using supplies; sorting, laundering (hand, machine, and dry clean); folding; ironing; storing; and mending.

    b. *Cleaning*—Obtaining and using supplies; picking up; putting away; vacuuming; sweeping and mopping floors; dusting; polishing; scrubbing; washing windows; cleaning mirrors; making beds; and removing trash and recyclables.

    c. *Meal Preparation/Cleanup*—Planning nutritious meals; preparing and serving food; opening and closing containers, cabinets, and drawers; using kitchen utensils and appliances; cleaning up and storing food safely.

    d. *Shopping*—Preparing shopping lists (grocery and other); selecting and purchasing items; selecting method of payment; and completing money transactions.

    e. *Money Management*—Budgeting, paying bills, and using bank systems.

    f. *Household Maintenance*—Maintaining home, yard, garden appliances, vehicles, and household items.

    g. *Safety Procedures*—Knowing and performing preventive and emergency procedures to maintain a safe environment and prevent injuries.

2. *Care of Others*—Providing for children, spouse, parents, pets, or others, such as giving physical care, nurturing, communicating, and using age-appropriate activities.

3. *Educational Activities*—Participating in a learning environment through school, community, or work-sponsored activities, such as exploring educational interests, attending to instruction, managing assignments, and contributing to group experiences.

4. *Vocational Activities*—Participating in work-related activities.

    a. *Vocational Exploration*—Determining aptitudes, developing interests and skills, and selecting appropriate vocational pursuits.

    b. *Job Acquisition*—Identifying and selecting work opportunities, and completing application and interview processes.

    c. *Work or Job Performance*—Performing job tasks in a timely and effective manner; incorporating necessary work behaviors.

    d. *Retirement Planning*—Determining aptitudes, developing interests and skills, and identifying appropriate avocational pursuits.

    e. *Volunteer Participation*—Performing unpaid activities for the benefit of selected individuals, groups, or causes.

C. *Play or Leisure Activities*—Intrinsically motivating activities for amusement, relaxation, spontaneous enjoyment, or self-expression.

1. *Play or Leisure Exploration*—Identifying interests, skills, opportunities, and appropriate play or leisure activities.

2. *Play or Leisure Performance*—Planning and participating in play or leisure activities; main-

taining a balance of play or leisure activities with work and productive activities, and activities of daily living; obtaining, utilizing, and maintaining equipment and supplies.

II. Performance Components

A. *Sensorimotor Components*—The ability to receive input, process information, and produce output.

1. *Sensory*

   a. *Sensory Awareness*—Receiving and differentiating sensory stimuli.

   b. *Sensory Processing*—Interpreting sensory stimuli.

   (1) *Tactile*—Interpreting light touch, pressure, temperature, pain, and vibration through skin contact/receptors.

   (2) *Proprioceptive*—Interpreting stimuli originating in muscles, joints, and other internal tissues to give information about the position of one body part in relation to another.

   (3) *Vestibular*—Interpreting stimuli from the inner ear receptors regarding head position and movement.

   (4) *Visual*—Interpreting stimuli through the eyes, including peripheral vision and acuity, awareness of color and pattern.

   (5) *Auditory*—Interpreting and localizing sounds, and discriminating background sounds.

   (6) *Gustatory*—Interpreting tastes.

   (7) *Olfactory*—Interpreting odors.

   c. *Perceptual Processing*—Organizing sensory input into meaningful patterns.

   (1) *Stereognosis*—Identifying objects through proprioception, cognition, and the sense of touch.

   (2) *Kinesthesia*—Identifying the excursion and direction of joint movement.

   (3) *Pain Response*—Interpreting noxious stimuli.

   (4) *Body Scheme*—Acquiring an internal awareness of the body and the relationship of body parts to each other.

   (5) *Right-Left Discrimination*—Differentiating one side of the body from the other.

   (6) *Form Constancy*—Recognizing forms and objects as the same in various environments, positions, and sizes.

   (7) *Position in Space*—Determining the spatial relationship of figures and objects to self or other forms and objects.

   (8) *Visual-Closure*—Identifying forms or objects from incomplete presentations.

   (9) *Figure Ground*—Differentiating between foreground and background forms and objects.

   (10) *Depth Perception*—Determining the relative distance between objects, figures, or landmarks and the observer, and changes in planes of surfaces.

   (11) *Spatial Relations*—Determining the position of objects relative to each other.

   (12) *Topographical Orientation*—Determining the location of objects and settings and the route to the location.

2. *Neuromusculoskeletal*

   a. *Reflex*—Eliciting an involuntary muscle response by sensory input.

   b. *Range of Motion*—Moving body parts through an arc.

   c. *Muscle Tone*—Demonstrating a degree of tension or resistance in a muscle at rest and in response to stretch.

   d. *Strength*—Demonstrating a degree of muscle power when movement is resisted, as with objects or gravity.

   e. *Endurance*—Sustaining cardiac, pulmonary, and musculoskeletal exertion over time.

   f. *Postural Control*—Using righting and equilibrium adjustments to maintain balance during functional movements.

   g. *Postural Alignment*—Maintaining biomechanical integrity among body parts.

   h. *Soft Tissue Integrity*—Maintaining anatomical and physiological condition of interstitial tissue and skin.

3. *Motor*

   a. *Gross Coordination*—Using large muscle groups for controlled, goal-directed movements.

   b. *Crossing the Midline*—Moving limbs and eyes across the midsagittal plane of the body.

   c. *Laterality*—Using a preferred unilateral body part for activities requiring a high level of skill.

d. *Bilateral Integration*—Coordinating both body sides during activity.

e. *Motor Control*—Using the body in functional and versatile movement patterns.

f. *Praxis*—Conceiving and planning a new motor act in response to an environmental demand.

g. *Fine Coordination/Dexterity*—Using small muscle groups for controlled movements, particularly in object manipulation.

h. *Visual-Motor Integration*—Coordinating the interaction of information from the eyes with body movement during activity.

i. *Oral-Motor Control*—Coordinating oropharyngeal musculature for controlled movements.

B. *Cognitive Integration and Cognitive Components*—The ability to use higher brain functions.

1. *Level of Arousal*—Demonstrating alertness and responsiveness to environmental stimuli.

2. *Orientation*—Identifying person, place, time, and situation.

3. *Recognition*—Identifying familiar faces, objects, and other previously presented materials.

4. *Attention Span*—Focusing on a task over time.

5. *Initiation of Activity*—Starting a physical or mental activity.

6. *Termination of Activity*—Stopping an activity at an appropriate time.

7. *Memory*—Recalling information after brief or long periods of time.

8. *Sequencing*—Placing information, concepts, and actions in order.

9. *Categorization*—Identifying similarities of and differences among pieces of environmental information.

10. *Concept Formation*—Organizing a variety of information to form thoughts and ideas.

11. *Spatial Operations*—Mentally manipulating the position of objects in various relationships.

12. *Problem Solving*—Recognizing a problem, defining a problem, identifying alternative plans, selecting a plan, organizing steps in a plan, implementing a plan, and evaluating the outcome.

13. *Learning*—Acquiring new concepts and behaviors.

14. *Generalization*—Applying previously learned concepts and behaviors to a variety of new situations.

C. *Psychosocial Skills and Psychological Components*—The ability to interact in society and to process emotions.

1. *Psychological*

a. *Values*—Identifying ideas or beliefs that are important to self and others.

b. *Interests*—Identifying mental or physical activities that create pleasure and maintain attention.

c. *Self-Concept*—Developing the value of the physical, emotional, and sexual self.

2. *Social*

a. *Role Performance*—Identifying, maintaining, and balancing functions one assumes or acquires in society (e.g., worker, student, parent, friend, religious participant).

b. *Social Conduct*—Interacting using manners, personal space, eye contact, gestures, active listening, and self-expression appropriate to one's environment.

c. *Interpersonal Skills*—Using verbal and nonverbal communication to interact in a variety of settings.

d. *Self-Expression*—Using a variety of styles and skills to express thoughts, feelings, and needs.

3. *Self-Management*

a. *Coping Skills*—Identifying and managing stress and related reactors.

b. *Time Management*—Planning and participating in a balance of self-care, work, leisure, and rest activities to promote satisfaction and health.

c. *Self-Control*—Modifying one's own behavior in response to environmental needs, demands, constraints, personal aspirations, and feedback from others.

III. Performance Contexts

Assessment of function in performance areas is greatly influenced by the contexts in which the individual must perform. Occupational therapy practitioners consider performance contexts when determining feasibility and appropriateness of interventions.

Occupational therapy practitioners may choose interventions based on an understanding of contexts, or may choose interventions directly aimed at altering the contexts to improve performance.

A. *Temporal Aspects*
1. *Chronological*—Individual's age.
2. *Developmental*—Stage or phase of maturation.
3. *Life Cycle*—Place in important life phases, such as career cycle, parenting cycle, or educational process.
4. *Disability Status*—Place in continuum of disability, such as acuteness of injury, chronicity of disability, or terminal nature of illness.

B. *Environmental Aspects*
1. *Physical*—Nonhuman aspects of contexts. Includes the accessibility to and performance within environments having natural terrain, plants, animals, buildings, furniture, objects, tools, or devices.
2. *Social*—Availability and expectations of significant individuals, such as spouse, friends, and caregivers. Also includes larger social groups which are influential in establishing norms, role expectations, and social routines.
3. *Cultural*—Customs, beliefs, activity patterns, behavior standards, and expectations accepted by the society of which the individual is a member. Includes political aspects, such as laws that affect access to resources and affirm personal rights. Also includes opportunities for education, employment, and economic support.

REFERENCES

American Occupational Therapy Association. (1979). *Occupational therapy output reporting system and uniform terminology for reporting occupational therapy services.* Rockville, MD: Author.

American Occupational Therapy Association. (1989). Uniform terminology for occupational therapy, Second edition. *American Journal of Occupational Therapy, 43,* 808-815.

American Occupational Therapy Association. (1993). Definition of occupational therapy practice for state regulation (Policy 5.3.1). *American Journal of Occupational Therapy, 47,* 1117-1121.

AUTHORS

The Terminology Task Force:
Winifred Dunn, PhD, OTR, FAOTA—Chairperson
Mary Foto, OTR, FAOTA
Jim Hinojosa, PhD, OTR, FAOTA
Barbara A. Boyt Schell, PhD, OTR/L, FAOTA
Linda Kohlman Thomson, MOT, OTR, OT(C), FAOTA
Sarah D. Hertfelder, MEd, MOT, OTR/L—Staff Liaison for The Commission on Practice
Jim Hinojosa, PhD, OTR, FAOTA—Chairperson

❖

Adopted by the Representative Assembly July 1994.

Note: This document replaces the following documents, all of which was rescinded by the 1994 Representative Assembly:

Occupational Therapy Product Output Reporting System (1979)
Uniform Terminology for Reporting Occupational Therapy Services, First Edition (1979)
Uniform Occupational Therapy Evaluation Checklist (1981)
Uniform Terminology for Occupational Therapy, Second Edition (1989)

UNIFORM TERMINOLOGY, THIRD EDITION

Application to Practice

INTRODUCTION

This document was developed to help occupational therapists apply *Uniform Terminology, Third Edition* to practice. The original grid format (Dunn, 1988) enabled occupational therapy practitioners to systematically identify deficit and strength areas of an individual and to select appropriate activities to address these areas in occupational therapy intervention (Dunn & McGourty, 1990). For the third edition, the profession is highlighting "Contexts" as another critical aspect of performance. A second grid provides therapy practitioners with a mechanism to consider the contextual features of performance in activities of daily living (ADL), work and productive activity, and play/leisure. "Performance Areas" and "Performance Components" (Figure A) focus on the individual. These features are embedded in the "Performance Contexts" (Figure B).

On the original grid (Dunn, 1988), the horizontal axis contains the Performance Areas of Activities of Daily Living, Work and Productive Activities, and Play or Leisure Activities (see Figure A). These Performance Areas are the functional outcomes occupational therapy addresses. The vertical axis contains the Performance Components, including Sensorimotor Components, Cognitive Components, and Psychosocial Components. The Performance Components are the skills and abilities that an individual uses to engage in the Performance Areas. During an occupational therapy assessment, the occupational therapy practitioner determines an individual's abilities and limitations in the Performance Components and how they affect the individual's functional outcomes in the Performance Areas.

Special Note: The first application document (Dunn & McGourty, 1989) describes how to use the original Uniform Terminology grid with a variety of individuals. It is quite useful to introduce these concepts. However, the Third Edition of Uniform Terminology contains some changes in the Performance Areas and Performance Components lists. Be sure to check for the terminology currently approved in the Third Edition before applying this information in current practice environments.

With the addition of Performance Contexts into Uniform Terminology, occupational therapy practitioners must consider how to interface what the individual wants to do (i.e., performance area) with the contextual features that may support or block performance. Figure B illustrates the interaction of Performance Areas and Performance Contexts as a model for therapists' planning.

The grid in Figure B can be used to analyze the contexts of performance for a particular individual. For example, when working with a toddler with a developmental disability who needs to learn to eat, the occupational therapy practitioner would consider all the Performance Contexts features as they might impact on this toddler's ability to master eating. Unlike the grid in Figure A, in which the occupational therapy practitioner selects both Performance Areas (i.e., what the individual wants or needs to do) and the Performance Component (i.e., a person's strengths and needs), in this grid (Figure B) the occupational therapy practitioner only selects the Performance Area. After the Performance Area is identified through collaboration with the individual and significant others, the occupational therapy practitioner considers ALL Performance Contexts features as they might impact on performance of the selected task.

Intervention Planning

Intervention planning occurs both within the general domain of concern of occupational therapy (i.e., Uniform Terminology) and by considering the profession's theoretical frames of reference that offer insights about how to approach the problem. In Figure A, the occupational therapy practitioner considers the Performance Areas that are of interest to the individual and the individual's strengths and concerns within the Performance Components. The intervention strategies would emerge from the cells on the grid that are placed at the intersection of the Performance Areas and the targeted Performance Components (strength and/or concern). For example, if a child needed to improve sensory processing and fine coordination for oral hygiene and grooming, an occupational therapy practitioner might select a sensory integrative frame of reference to create intervention strategies, such as adding textures to handles and teaching the child

PERFORMANCE AREAS

ACTIVITIES OF DAILY LIVING
Grooming
Oral Hygiene
Bathing/Showering
Toilet Hygiene
Personal Device Care
Dressing
Feeding and Eating
Medication Routine
Health Maintenance
Socialization
Functional Communication
Functional Mobility
Community Mobility
Emergency Response
Sexual Expression
WORK AND PRODUCTIVE ACTIVITIES
Home Management
Care of Others
Educational Activities
Vocational Activities
PLAY OR LEISURE ACTIVITIES
Play or Leisure Exploration
Play or Leisure Performance

PERFORMANCE COMPONENTS

A. SENSORIMOTOR COMPONENT
  1. Sensory
    a. Sensory Awareness
    b. Sensory Processing
      (1) Tactile
      (2) Proprioceptive
      (3) Vestibular
      (4) Visual
      (5) Auditory
      (6) Gustatory
      (7) Olfactory
    c. Perceptual Processing
      (1) Stereognosis
      (2) Kinesthesia
      (3) Pain Response
      (4) Body Scheme
      (5) Right-Left Discrimination
      (6) Form Constancy
      (7) Position in Space
      (8) Visual-Closure
      (9) Figure Ground
      (10) Depth Perception
      (11) Spatial Relations
      (12) Topographical Orientation
  2. Neuromusculoskeletal
    a. Reflex
    b. Range of Motion
    c. Muscle Tone
    d. Strength
    e. Endurance
    f. Postural Control
    g. Postural Alignment
    h. Soft Tissue Integrity

Figure A. Uniform Terminology Grid (Performance Areas and Performance Components).

Figure A (continued)

PERFORMANCE AREAS

Column headers:
- ACTIVITIES OF DAILY LIVING: Grooming, Oral Hygiene, Bathing/Showering, Toilet Hygiene, Personal Device Care, Dressing, Feeding and Eating, Medication Routine, Health Maintenance, Socialization, Functional Communication, Functional Mobility, Community Mobility, Emergency Response, Sexual Expression
- WORK AND PRODUCTIVE ACTIVITIES: Home Management, Care of Others, Educational Activities, Vocational Activities
- PLAY OR LEISURE ACTIVITIES: Play or Leisure Exploration, Play or Leisure Performance

Row labels:

3. Motor
  a. Gross Coordination
  b. Crossing the Midline
  c. Laterality
  d. Bilateral Integration
  e. Motor Control
  f. Praxis
  g. Fine Coordination/Dexterity
  h. Visual-Motor Integration
  i. Oral-Motor Control

B. COGNITIVE INTEGRATION AND COGNITIVE COMPONENTS
  1. Level of Arousal
  2. Orientation
  3. Recognition
  4. Attention Span
  5. Initiation of Activity
  6. Termination of Activity
  7. Memory
  8. Sequencing
  9. Categorization
  10. Concept Formation
  11. Spatial Operations
  12. Problem Solving
  13. Learning
  14. Generalization

C. PSYCHOSOCIAL SKILLS AND PSYCHOLOGICAL COMPONENTS
  1. Psychological
    a. Values
    b. Interests
    c. Self-Concept
  2. Social
    a. Role Performance
    b. Social Conduct
    c. Interpersonal Skills
    d. Self-Expression
  3. Self-Management
    a. Coping Skills
    b. Time Management
    c. Self-Control

Figure A (continued). Uniform Terminology Grid (Performance Areas and Performance Components).

Figure B. Uniform Terminology Grid (Performance Areas and Performance Contexts).

sand and bean digging games. Dunn and McGourty (1989) discuss this in more detail.

When using Figure B, the occupational therapy practitioner considers the Performance Contexts features in relation to the desired Performance Area. The occupational therapy practitioner would analyze the individual's temporal, physical, social, and cultural contexts to determine the relevance of particular interventions. For example, if the child mentioned above was a member of a family in which having messy hands from sand play was unacceptable, the occupational therapy practitioner would consider alternate strategies that are more compatible with their lifestyle. For example, perhaps the family would be more interested in developing puppet play. This would still provide the child with opportunities to experience the textures of various puppets and the hand movements required to manipulate the puppets in play context, without adding the messiness of sand. When occupational therapy practitioners consider contexts, interventions become more relevant and applicable to individual's lives.

CASE EXAMPLE 1

Sophie, a 75-year-old woman who was widowed 3 years ago, is recovering from a cerebral vascular accident and has been transferred from an acute care unit to an inpatient medical rehabilitation unit. Prior to her admission, she was living in a small house in an isolated location and has no family living nearby. She was driving independently and frequently ran errands for her friends. She is adamant in her goal to return to her home after discharge. All of her friends are quite elderly and are not able to provide many resources for support.

Sophie and the team collaborated to identify her goals. Sophie decided that she wanted to be able to meet her daily needs with little or no assistance. Almost all of the Performance Areas are critical in order to achieve the outcome of community living in her own home. Being able to cook all of her meals, bathe independently, and have alternative transportation available is necessary. Because of their significant impact on the patient's function in the Performance Areas, some of the Performance Components that may need to be addressed are figure ground, muscle tone, postural control, fine coordination, memory, and self-management.

In the selection of occupational therapy interventions, it is critical to analyze the elements of Performance Contexts for the individual. The physical and social elements of her home environment do not support returning home without modifications to her home and additional social supports being established. Railings must be added to the front steps, provision of and instruction in the use of a tub seat, and instruction in the use of specialized transportation may need to occur. If this same individual had been living in an apartment in a retirement community prior to her CVA, the contexts of performance would support a return home with fewer environmental modifications being needed. Being independent in cooking might not be necessary due to meals being provided, and the bathroom might already be accessible and safe. If the individual had friends and family available, the social support network might already be established to assist with shopping and transportation needs. The occupational therapy interventions would be different due to the contexts in which the individual will be performing. Interventions must be selected with the impact of the Performance Contexts as an essential element.

CASE EXAMPLE 2

Malcolm is a 9-year-old boy who has a learning disability which causes him to have a variety of problems in school. His teachers complain that he is difficult to manage in the classroom. Some of the Performance Components that may need to be addressed are his self-control such as interrupting, difficulty sitting during instruction, and difficulty with peer relations. Other children avoid him on the playground because he doesn't follow rules, doesn't play fair, and tends to anger quickly when confronted. The performance component impairment with concept formation is reflected in his sloppy and disorganized classroom assignments.

The critical elements of the Performance Contexts are the temporal aspect of age-appropriateness of his behavior and the social environmental aspect of his immature socialization. The significant cultural and temporal aspects of his family are that they place a high premium on athletic prowess.

The occupational therapy practitioner intervenes in several ways to address his behavior in the school environment. The occupational therapy practitioner focuses on structuring the classroom environment and facilitating consistent behavioral expectations for Malcolm by educational personnel. She also consults with the teachers to develop ways to structure activities which will support his ability to relate to other children in a positive way.

In contrast, another child with similar learning disabilities, but who is 12 years old and in the 7th grade might have different concerns. Elements of the Performance Contexts are the temporal aspect of the age-appropriateness of his behavior; and the social environment context of school where "bullying" behavior is unacceptable and in which completing assignments is expected. In addressing the cultural Performance Contexts the occupational therapy practitioner recognizes from meeting the parents that they have only average expectation for academic performance but value athletic accomplishments.

Since teachers at his school consider completion of home assignments to be part of average performance, the occupational therapy practitioner works with the child and parents on time management and reinforcement strategies to meet this expectation. After consultation with the coach, she works with the father to create activities to improve his athletic abilities. When occupational therapy practitioners consider family values as part of the contexts of performance, different intervention priorities may emerge.

Authors

The Terminology Task Force:
Winifred Dunn, PhD, OTR, FAOTA—
Chairperson
Mary Foto, OTR, FAOTA
Jim Hinojosa, PhD, OTR, FAOTA
Barbara A. Boyt Schell, PhD, OTR/L, FAOTA
Linda Kohlman Thomson, MOT, OTR, OT(C),
FAOTA
Sarah D. Hertfelder, MEd, MOT, OTR/L—
Staff Liaison for the Commission on
Practice, 1994
Jim Hinojosa, PhD, OTR, FAOTA—Chair-
person

❖

Note: This document replaces the 1989
Application of Uniform Terminology to Practice that
accompanied the *Uniform Terminology for
Occupational Therapy, Second Edition.*

Appendix D

BLANK STUDENT WORKSHEETS

Form I

ACTIVITY AWARENESS FORM

Student: _____   Date: _____
Activity: _____
Course: _____

Directions: Reflecting on the activity just performed, complete the following sentences with the first words that come to mind.

1. During this activity I was thinking about...

2. While doing this activity I felt...

3. In doing this activity, the parts of my body I remember using were...

4. To do this activity I need to (mentally, emotionally, physically)...

5. When I do this activity again I will...

6. From doing this activity I became aware of...

Form 2

ACTION IDENTIFICATION FORM

Student: _____   Date: _____

Activity: _____

Course: _____

Directions: Select an activity and list the major actions (in sequence) required for you to perform this activity in 10 steps or less. Repeat the exercise after observing someone else perform the same activity. Use the "Do-What-How" format.

Observations of Self	Observations of Another

Form 3

ACTIVITY ANALYSIS FOR EXPECTED PERFORMANCE

Student: _____   Date: _____

Activity: _____

Course: _____

SECTION 1: ACTIVITY SUMMARY

Directions: Respond to the following in list format.

1. Name of Activity

2. Brief Description of Activity

3. Tools/Equipment (non-expendable), Cost, and Source

4. Materials/Supplies (expendable), Cost, and Source

5. Space/Environmental Requirements

6. Sequence of Major Steps (in 10 steps or less; specify time required to complete each step)

7. Precautions (review "Sequence of Major Steps")

8. Special Considerations (age appropriateness, educational requirements, cultural relevance, gender identification, other)

9. Acceptable Criteria for Completed Project

SECTION 2: ANALYZING OCCUPATIONAL PERFORMANCE AREAS, COMPONENTS, AND CONTEXTS

Part I. Performance Areas

A. Activities of Daily Living
   1. Grooming

   2. Oral Hygiene

   3. Bathing/Showering

   4. Toilet Hygiene

   5. Personal Device Care

   6. Dressing

7. Feeding and Eating

8. Medication Routine

9. Health Maintenance

10. Socialization

11. Functional Communication

12. Functional Mobility

13. Community Mobility

14. Emergency Response

15. Sexual Expression

B. Work and Productive Activities
   1. Home Management
      a. Clothing Care

      b. Cleaning

      c. Meal Preparation/Cleanup

      d. Shopping

      e. Money Management

      f. Household Maintenance

      g. Safety Procedures

   2. Care of Others

   3. Educational Activities

   4. Vocational Activities
      a. Vocational Exploration

      b. Job Acquisition

      c. Work or Job Performance

      d. Retirement Planning

      e. Volunteer Participation

C. Play or Leisure Activities
   1. Play or Leisure Exploration

   2. Play or Leisure Performance

Part II. Performance Components

A. Sensorimotor Components
   1. Sensory
      a. Sensory Awareness

      b. Sensory Processing
         (1) Tactile

         (2) Proprioceptive

         (3) Vestibular

         (4) Visual

         (5) Auditory

         (6) Gustatory

         (7) Olfactory

      c. Perceptual Processing
         (1) Stereognosis

         (2) Kinesthesia

         (3) Pain Response

         (4) Body Scheme

         (5) Right-Left Discrimination

         (6) Form Constancy

         (7) Position in Space

         (8) Visual-Closure

         (9) Figure Ground

         (10) Depth Perception

         (11) Spatial Relations

         (12) Topographical Orientation

   2. Neuromusculoskeletal
      a. Reflex

      b. Range of Motion

      c. Muscle Tone

    d. Strength

    e. Endurance

    f. Postural Control

    g. Postural Alignment

    h. Soft Tissue Integrity

3. Motor
    a. Gross Coordination

    b. Crossing the Midline

    c. Laterality

    d. Bilateral Integration

    e. Motor Control

    f. Praxis

    g. Fine Coordination/Dexterity

    h. Visual-Motor Integration

    i. Oral-Motor Control

B. Cognitive Integration and Cognitive Components
1. Level of Arousal

2. Orientation

3. Recognition

4. Attention Span

5. Initiation of Activity

6. Termination of Activity

7. Memory

8. Sequencing

9. Categorization

10. Concept Formation

11. Spatial Operations

12. Problem Solving

13. Learning

14. Generalization

C. Psychosocial Skills and Psychological Components
  1. Psychological
     a. Values

     b. Interests

     c. Self-Concept

  2. Social
     a. Role Performance

     b. Social Conduct

     c. Interpersonal Skills

     d. Self-Expression

  3. Self-Management
     a. Coping Skills

     b. Time Management

     c. Self-Control

Part III. Performance Contexts

A. Temporal Aspects
  1. Chronological

  2. Developmental

  3. Life Cycle

  4. Disability Status

B. Environmental Aspects
  1. Physical

  2. Social

  3. Cultural

Form 4

ACTIVITY ANALYSIS FOR THERAPEUTIC INTERVENTION

Student: _____   Date: _____

Activity: _____

Course: _____

SECTION 1: ACTIVITY DESCRIPTION

A. Provide a brief description of activity.

B. Identify major steps.

SECTION 2: THERAPEUTIC QUALITIES

A. Energy Patterns—Describe the required energy level in terms of light, moderate, or heavy work patterns and provide an explanation for the level specified.

B. Activity Patterns—Indicate the patterns of the activity expected for successful completion of the activity.

   1. Structural/Methodical/Orderly

   2. Repetitive

   3 Expressive/Creative/Projective

   4. Tactile
      a. Contact with others (e.g., hands-on, stand by assist)

      b. Materials (e.g., pliable, sensual)

      c. Equipment (e.g., size, manageability, shape)

SECTION 3: THERAPEUTIC APPLICATION

Part I. Population

Discuss for whom and in what way increased occupational performance can be derived from the use of this activity. Consider the sensorimotor, cognitive, and psychosocial aspects. Identify any contraindications.

Part II. Gradation

Describe ways to grade this activity in terms of:

1. Activity Sequence, Duration, and/or the Activity Procedures

2. Working Position of the Individual

3. Tools
   a. Position

   b. Size

   c. Shape

   d. Weight

   e. Texture

4. Materials
   a. position

   b. size

   c. shape

   d. weight

   e. texture

5. Nature/Degree of Interpersonal Contact

6. Extent of Tactile, Verbal, or Visual Cues Used by Practitioner During Activity

7. The Teaching-Learning Environment

Part III. Therapeutic Modifications

Indicate ways in which this activity may be changed to increase occupational performance. State your reasoning. Write "n/a" if not applicable. Definitions for the following terms can be found in Appendix B, *Uniform Terminology for Reporting Occupational Therapy Services, First Edition*, "Therapeutic Adaptations" and "The Guide to O.T. Practice," AOTA, 1999.

A. Therapeutic Adaptations
 1. Orthotic Devices

 2. Prosthetic Devices

 3. Assistive Technology and Adaptive Devices
  a. Architectural Modification

  b. Environmental Modification

  c. Tool and Equipment Modification (low tech: e.g., reacher; high tech: e.g., computer control devices)

  d. Wheelchair Modification

 4. Prevention
  a. Energy Conservation
   (1) Energy-Saving Procedures

   (2) Activity Restriction

   (3) Work Simplification

   (4) Time Management

   (5) Environmental Organization

b. Joint Protection/Body Mechanics
   (1) Using Proper Body Mechanics

   (2) Avoiding Static/Deforming Postures

   (3) Avoiding Excessive Weight-Bearing

c. Positioning

d. Balance of Performance Areas to Facilitate Health and Well-being
   (1) Enhancement of Occupational Performance Areas

   (2) Satisfaction of Client and/or Caregiver

   (3) Quality of Life

Form 5
CLIENT-ACTIVITY CORRELATION FORM

Student: _____   Date: _____

Activity: _____

Course: _____

1. Client Profile and Referral

2. Intervention Goals

    a. Long-Term Goals

    b. Short-Term Goals

3. Goal-Directed Purposeful Activity Description

4. Activity Preparation

    a. Review Goals, Describe Practitioner's Role

    b. Personnel Required to do the Preparation

c. Required Preparation Time

d. Required Place and Space

e. Materials

f. Equipment

g. Safety Precautions for Personnel

5. Activity Implementation

   a. Personnel

   b. Setting and Location

   c. Space Required

   d. Environment

e. Materials

f. Equipment: Assistive Devices and Adaptations Included

g. Required Intervention Time

h. Safety Precautions for Client

6. Client-Practitioner Activity Sequence (10 action steps or less)

7. Uniform Terminology Documentation

INDEX